ORDER FORM

Send book(s) to:

Name _____

Address _____

City _____ State _____ Zip _____

PRICES:

    1 @ $ 9.95 each
    2 @ $19.90
  3–10 @ $ 8.95 each
 11–20 @ $ 8.25 each
 21–30 @ $ 7.55 each
 31–50 @ $ 6.85 each
51–100 @ $ 6.50 each

Price includes postage & handling.

Quantity _____ @ $ _____

TOTAL ENCLOSED _____

PREPAYMENT REQUIRED.
PLEASE PAY IN U.S. FUNDS.
OUTSIDE U.S.A., SEND ADDITIONAL $1.00/BOOK.
ALLOW 4–6 WEEKS FOR DELIVERY.

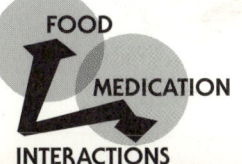

Enclose with your check or money order in an envelope.

MAIL TO:

FOOD-MEDICATION INTERACTIONS

P.O. Box 44033   or   P.O. Box 26464
Phoenix, Arizona 85064   Tempe, Arizona 85285

FOOD MEDICATION INTERACTIONS

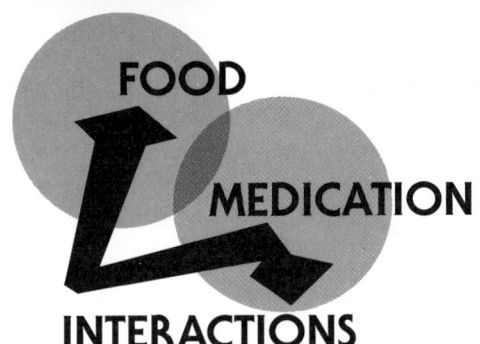

6th Edition

by

Dorothy E. Powers, R.D.
Ann O. Moore, M.S., R.D.

Published & Distributed by Food Medication Interactions
P.O. Box 44033, Phoenix, Arizona 85064

© 1988 by Dorothy E. Powers, R.D.
    and Ann O. Moore, M.S., R.D.

First Edition, December, 1978
Second Edition, May, 1979
Third Edition, May, 1981
Fourth Edition, October, 1983
Fifth Edition, March, 1986
Sixth Edition, August, 1988, Second Printing, January, 1989.
All publication and reproduction rights reserved and prohibited to others.

ISBN 0-9606164-2-X
Printed in USA

EDITORS: Linda K. McCoy, Pharm.D.
Manager of Clinical Services
Department of Pharmacy Services
Good Samaritan Medical Center
1111 E. McDowell Road
Phoenix, Arizona

Christine Hamilton Smith, Ph.D., R.D., Professor
Food Science and Nutrition,
Home Economics Department
California State University
Northridge
Northridge, California

We are indebted to the Editors for their constructive and skillful editing of this material; for their contribution of resources, critical comments, and expertise; and for the excellent suggestions regarding the clinical orientation of this material.

ACKNOWLEDGMENTS

We are most thankful for the substantial contributions and continued support of all the health professionals who have aided us in this endeavor. Those who have provided special assistance in the preparation of this edition include:

G. H. Powers, M.D., J. M. Powers, M.D., J. L. Powers, M.D., Catherine Corak, R.D., Sue Zevan, R.D., Pamela Gallagher, M.D.

In doing this Sixth Edition, we appreciate Celeste Wilson-Stone giving unsparingly of her computer skills and talents.

DEP & AOM

PREFACE

The ever increasing interest in the interactions between food/nutrients and medications has stimulated the publication of this edition. The Joint Commission on the Accreditation of Hospitals has made dietitians responsible for monitoring the occurrence of drug-nutrient interactions in acute care hospitals and for counseling patients about the best means to prevent these events (40). The sixth edition is a specially designed pocket-sized book, containing medications most commonly used. Up-to-date information is provided in a concise form. Drugs are listed alphabetically by generic and trade names for easy reference.

Prior to use, readers are urged to review the Guide to the Use of This Book and the Table of Contents to familiarize themselves with the style and organization of this book.

Changes in nutritional status can happen through one or more possible mechanisms. Cost effective nutritional care can be enhanced by recognizing the changes drugs make on nutritional status. It is hoped that the use of this edition by all health care professionals will contribute to quality care through improved drug utilization and patient compliance and comfort.

World-wide distribution has been a source of satisfaction. Comments and recommendations concerning the book and its contents are encouraged.

Contact the authors for specific references at P.O. Box 44033, Phoenix, Arizona 85064. (602) 251-2465, a message center.

GUIDE TO THE USE OF THIS BOOK

A specific format is followed for each medication:
1. **Medications** are listed alphabetically by generic name *(italics)* and by trade name (**bold**).
2. **Classification** indicates the purpose of the drug.
3. **Dietary/Related Significances** appear under the generic name. Exception: Medications containing multiple drugs may appear under the trade name. ''See listing for . . .'' denotes that the effects are similar, although composition of the drug is different.
   A. **Drug** (when and how to take drug) refers to the proper oral administration of the medicine and may relate to specific food and fluid intake if this effect is clinically important.
   B. **Diet** includes specific and known dietary suggestions, including the interactive effects of vitamin/mineral supplements.
   C. **Nutr** (Nutrition) refers to implications, alterations in nutrients, e.g. B_{12} absorption.
   D. **GI** (Gastrointestinal) pertains to stomach, intestines, colon, e.g. constipation, flatulence, n&v.
   E. **S/Cond** (Special Conditions) refers to a potential reaction alert, e.g. diabetic: prolonged use ↓ CHO tolerance. Limit alcohol: 1–2oz with physician's permission.
   F. **Metab/Phys** (Metabolic/Physiological) pertains to possible changes in function, e.g. anemias, edema, osteomalacia.
   G. **Other** includes effects relating to possible alterations in food consumption, e.g. ↑ appetite for sweets, dry mouth, tremors, fatigue, headache.
   H. **Blood/Serum, Urinary** indicates that medications may alter laboratory values.
4. Clinically significant changes are underlined.
5. When the medication contains **pharmacologically active substances,** e.g., alcohol, sugars, sodium, potassium, caffeine, tartrazine, sulfites, they are listed when the information is available.
6. Selected References are noted by number, e.g. ''Limit Pyr to 10mg/day.[13]''

CONTACT THE AUTHORS FOR OTHER SPECIFIC REFERENCES AT: P.O. BOX 26464, TEMPE, ARIZONA, 85285 or P.O. BOX 44033, PHOENIX, ARIZONA 85064. (602) 251-2465, A MESSAGE CENTER.

CONTACT YOUR PHARMACIST or REGISTERED DIETITIAN IF THERE IS ANY CONCERN ABOUT A FOOD-MEDICATION INTERACTION.

ABBREVIATIONS and SYMBOLS

ADH	antidiuretic hormone	mEq	milliequivalents
alk phos	alkaline phosphatase	Mg	magnesium
Al	aluminum	mg	milligram
$\bar{c}$	with	ml	milliliter (also, cc)
Ca	calcium	Mn	manganese
cal	calorie	N	nitrogen
cap	capsule	Na	sodium
CHO	carbohydrate	n & v	nausea & vomiting
chol	cholesterol	Nia	niacin
Cl	chloride	NSAI	non-steroidal anti-inflammatory
CNS	central nervous system	P	phosphorus
↓	decreased (low)	(P)	phosphate
e.g.	for example	PCM	protein-calorie malnutrition
ETOH	ethanol	Pyr	pyridoxine
Fe	iron	Rib	riboflavin
Fol	folacin	tab	tablet
GI	gastrointestinal	TG	triglyceride
G6PD	glucose-6-phosphate dehydrogenase	Thi	thiamin
HCTZ	hydrochlorothiazide	Vit A	vitamin A
hr	hour	Vit B-6	vitamin B_6
H_2O	water	Vit B-12	vitamin B_{12}
↑	increased (high)	Vit C	vitamin C (ascorbic acid)
IU	international units	Vit D	vitamin D
K	potassium	Vit E	vitamin E
kg	kilograms	Vit K	vitamin K
L	liter	wt	weight
MAOI	monoamine oxidase inhibitor	Zn	zinc
μg	micrograms	$\bar{s}$	without
MCT	medium chain triglyceride	U	unit

*Abbreviations for Laboratory Values are found in Table p. 217.

TABLE OF CONTENTS

1. Preface	4
2. Guide to the Use of This Book	5
3. Abbreviations and Symbols	6
4. Table of Contents	7
5. Introduction	8
6. Mechanisms of Interactions	10
7. Dietary Suggestions	27
8. Guidelines to Counseling Medicated Patients	32
9. Food-Medication Interactions	35
10. Tables: A. Laboratory Values	217
B. Comparison of Height-Weight Tables	228
C. Segmental Weights for Limbs, Calculation of Desirable Body Weight	229
D. Adult Height-Weight Ranges	230
E. Caffeine Content of Selected Foods & Beverages	231
F. Herbal Teas: Caution	232
G. Food Sources of Oxalates	233
H. Pressor Agents	234
I. Patient Counseling	235
J. Goitrogenic Foods	236
K. Vitamin K in Selected Foods & Beverages	236
L. Tabulation of pH and Acid Content	237
M. Foods Potentially Causing Changes in Urinary pH	238
N. Salt Substitutes	239
O. Physical Signs of Malnutrition	240
11. References	244
12. Additional References	247

INTRODUCTION TO FOOD-MEDICATION INTERACTIONS

Medications can be affected by food or can affect nutritional status. The question of drugs, nutrition and their interrelationship becomes pertinent, since nutrition plays a vital role in the expanding medical services available for patients.

Vulnerability to drug-induced nutritional deficiencies is greatest in the elderly, the chronically-ill, in the growing child, in pregnancy and lactation, and in anyone with marginal or inadequate nutrient intake. At special risk are those patients who are under long-term drug therapy or stress. In children, dosages of drugs are usually decreased due to immaturity of drug metabolism in the liver. The newborn infant requires drug administration based on biological maturity, gestational age, birth weight, and presence and extent of disease. Safe use in pregnancy has not been established for most drugs, relative to the possible adverse effects on fetal development. In lactation, many drugs may distribute readily into breast milk.

The impact of drugs on nutritional status and the effects of food, special diets and dietary habits on drug action have to be evaluated in patients on an individual basis. A myriad of coparticipants (age-related nutrient requirements, dietary habits, gender, reproductive status, need for therapeutic diets, the underlying illness, polypharmacy, nutrient supplements, drug dosage, duration of drug therapy, alcohol use) can, also, impinge upon the overall health status of the patient. It is, therefore, critical for health professionals to be aware of all facets of potential interactions among foods, nutrients and drugs that can complicate dietary and drug therapy in the individual patient.

Hematological disorders are of particular concern in nutritional care. These blood dyscrasias include nutritional anemia, platelet dysfunction, leukopenia or agranulocytosis. Treatments vary and <u>may</u> include diet evaluation and therapy. However, the dietitian should be aware that diet therapy may play no supportive role in the treatment of some of these conditions.

Please note that food and drug effects are possibilities documented. Our reporting does not imply these effects happen to all. The effects of drugs in the same classification with different chemical structures can result in similar significances.

To enable the dietitian, food service supervisor, and nursing staff to adjust dietary procedures to the drug regimen in order to give optimal patient care, the following information provides a review of how medications may affect nutrients or how drug actions can be affected by food or alcohol. Also, included are possible alcohol-drug interactions, guidelines for counseling medicated patients and dietary suggestions to aid in the relief of nutrition related side effects of drugs.

Users of the *Food-Medication Interactions* pocketbook are urged to review this information to facilitate conceptual understanding of the mechanisms of interactions between medications and food, nutrients, alcohol, and vitamin/mineral supplements.

MECHANISMS OF INTERACTIONS
EFFECTS OF DRUGS ON NUTRITIONAL STATUS

I. MODIFIED FOOD INTAKE

As a Result of:	Example
A. Taste/Smell Dysfunction	Some drugs may be secreted into the saliva and produce an unpleasant taste in the mouth, or may cause an unpleasant aftertaste. Some drugs may themselves be unpalatable or may have a disagreeable texture (potassium preparations, cholestyramine, penicillin, metronidazole). Altered taste receptor function may also be a factor in taste disorders (captopril, penicillamine). Decreased olfactory receptor response may occur from chronic use of antihistamines or bronchodilators.
B. Dry Mouth	Dry mouth may result from various drugs such as the diuretics or those with anticholinergic action (phenothiazines, tricyclic antidepressants).
C. Gastric Irritation	Almost any drug taken orally has the potential for irritating the gastric mucosa, e.g. analgesics.

D. Bezoars — Formed from concretions of poorly crushed and dissolved tablets (sucralfate, aluminum hydroxide gel, antacid tablets, iron tablets, cholestyramine) or from a compact mass of matted plant fibers or other food matter (phytobezoar). Intragastric mass may form in some patients with achlorhydria and in patients with surgically-induced alterations in gastric function, symptoms of which range from epigastric fullness to attacks of pain, nausea and vomiting. May also cause gastric outlet obstruction and other serious gastrointestinal disorders. Patient may be advised to follow a low-fiber, anti-bezoar diet.[43]

E. Appetite Suppression — Metabolic influences, nausea, GI distress, e.g. anorexiants, antineoplastics.

F. Appetite Stimulation — Metabolic influences or renewed awareness of food, e.g. long-term use of antidepressants, antipsychotics.

G. Nausea/Vomiting — Disagreeable symptoms that may occur singly or concurrently and from a wide variety of drugs (levodopa, propoxyphene, sulfasalazine, antineoplastics). Drugs, such as some digitalis derivatives, can directly stimulate the chemoreceptor trigger zone and initiate vomiting. Nausea and vomiting can also result from drug-induced irritative stimuli in the gastrointestinal tract itself.

II. MODIFIED NUTRIENT ABSORPTION

As a Result of:	Example
A. GI pH altered	Chronic use of antacids may increase pH, thiamin unstable in basic pH: hence thiamin deficiency.
B. Bile acid activity	Antihyperlipemics bind bile acids: malabsorption of fat and some fat-soluble nutrients.
C. GI motility altered	Laxative and cathartics may induce hyperperistalsis: decreased glucose absorption.
D. Intestinal mucosal coating	Mineral oil acts as a physical barrier and lipid solvent: impaired absorption of fat-soluble vitamins and other nutrients.
E. Enzyme inhibition	Some antibiotics may inhibit intestinal disaccharidases or folate conjugase: fecal nutrient loss and diarrhea.
F. Mucosal cell wall damage	The antimitotic activity of antigout agents and some antineoplastic agents causes structural damage to the intestinal mucosa.
G. Insoluble nutrient complexes	Aluminum hydroxide gel binds phosphate or iron as poorly absorbed insoluble complexes.

III. MODIFIED NUTRIENT METABOLISM

As a Result of: Example

A. Vitamin antagonism

Isoniazid, cycloserine, penicillamine and hydralazine impair normal metabolism of vitamin B_6.

B. Induced vitamin inactivation

Anticonvulsant (phenytoin) induction of hepatic microsomal enzymes may accelerate the conversion of vitamin D to inactive derivatives. (Effect may also be due to altered metabolism of vitamin K.)

IV. MODIFIED NUTRIENT EXCRETION

A. Urinary loss of nutrients

Hydrocortisone or potassium-depleting diuretics increase potassium excretion.

B. Fecal loss of nutrients

Prolonged use of laxatives may produce electrolyte imbalance.

EFFECTS OF FOODS/NUTRIENTS ON DRUG RESPONSE

I. MODIFIED DRUG ABSORPTION

As a Result of:	Example
A. Gastric emptying time, delayed	Food in the stomach delays rate of gastric emptying and may enhance drug bioavailability (nitrofurantoin).
B. First-pass metabolism, altered	Ingestion of food may reduce first-pass metabolism (biotransformation) and increase drug bioavailability (propranolol).
C. Dissolution	Fatty meals enhance dissolution of griseofulvin, thus increasing drug absorption.
D. Drug-nutrient chelation	Impaired tetracycline absorption may occur when concurrently taken with foods or beverages containing calcium or with iron-rich or iron- or calcium-fortified foods. Insoluble chelates will also be formed from interactions between tetracycline and other di- or trivalent cations (eg., zinc, magnesium).
E. Competitive inhibition	Competition for absorptive sites in the intestine by dietary amino acids interferes with the bioavailability of levodopa.

II. MODIFIED DRUG ACTION

As a Result of:	Example
A. Drug antagonism	A large intake of foods rich in vitamin K may inhibit hypoprothrombinemic response to oral anticoagulants. See Table p. 236.
B. Urinary excretion, altered	Low-sodium diet (after drug stabilization) may cause renal reabsorption of lithium and result in accumulation of drug to toxic levels.
	Excessive intake of alkaline-ash foods may enhance tubular reabsorption of quinidine (antiarrhythmic agent) by increasing urinary pH.

EFFECTS OF INTERACTIONS BETWEEN DRUGS AND VITAMINS/MINERAL SUPPLEMENTS

I. DECREASED VITAMIN/MINERAL ABSORPTION

As a Result of:	Example
A. Bile acid activity, altered	Aluminum-containing antacids (aluminum hydroxide) may precipitate bile acids, thus decreasing absorption of fat-soluble vitamins (vitamin A).
	Concurrent use of bile acid sequestrants (cholestyramine, colestipol) may inhibit the absorption of Vit A.
B. Nutrient-drug chelation	Concurrent intake of tetracycline with calcium, iron, zinc, and magnesium supplements may result in the formation of nonabsorbable complexes, thus impairing both drug and mineral absorption.
	Concurrent intake decreases the bioavailability of both phenytoin and calcium due to the formation of nonabsorbable complexes, thus impairing both drug and mineral absorption.

II. DECREASED DRUG ABSORPTION
As a Result of:

	Example
A. Nutrient-drug chelation	See above.
	Iron preparations may inhibit the absorption of penicillamine, thus impairing the therapeutic effects of the drug.

III. MODIFIED DRUG ACTION
As a Result of:

	Example
A. Deranged calcium metabolism	Hypervitaminosis D-induced hypercalcemia may enhance the toxic effects of digitalis glycosides.
B. Inhibition of vitamin K absorption or action (?)	Large doses of vitamin E may increase hypoprothrombinemic effect of oral anticoagulants (warfarin).
C. Biotransformation, altered	Folacin may increase the formation and excretion of hydroxylated metabolites of phenytoin.

IV: OTHER INTERACTIONS:

Vitamin/ Mineral Supplement	Drug	Effect
Vitamin A	isotretinoin	Additive toxic effects may result from combination therapy.
Vitamin C	warfarin	Megadoses may interfere with drug absorption and decrease prothrombin time.
Vitamin D	calcium carbonate	Concurrent use and long term therapy may result in milk-alkali syndrome.
Calcium	hydrochlorothiazide	Concurrent use may result in hypercalcemia.

PHARMACOLOGIC INTERACTIONS BETWEEN DRUGS AND NON-NUTRIENTS IN FOOD

Several foods contain components with pharmacologic activity that are not expressed under normal circumstances. Also, a number of bioactive food substances and dyes possess pharmacologic activity that may agonize or antagonize the pharmacologic activity of certain drugs.

A. Tyramine and other pressor agents

The combination of monoamine oxidase inhibitors and tyramine-containing foods may cause dangerous increases in blood pressure. See Table p. 234.

B. Caffeine

Caffeine belongs to a family of chemical compounds called xanthines. Caffeine and its related compounds act as central nervous system and heart muscle stimulants, diuretics, and muscle relaxants. Intake of 200 mg caffeine may be considered as a pharmacologic amount. See Table p. 231.

C. Tartrazine

FDA requires the listing of Yellow Dye No. 5 (tartrazine) color additive, as an ingredient when present in foods and drugs. The information will be useful in counseling tartrazine-allergic patients.

D. Oxalates

Oxalate-containing foods need to be avoided during drug treatment of specific disorders. Certain types of kidney stones contain large amounts. See Table p. 233.

E. Monosodium Glutamate

"Chinese restaurant syndrome" mimics angina in sensitive patients. Those on long-term anti-hypertensive therapy should be cautious about consuming large quantities.

F. Licorice glycyrrhizic acid

Natural extract of glycyrrhiza root used in "natural" licorice candies may antagonize the action of diuretics and drugs and add to the mineralocorticoid effects of the adrenocorticoids. Two or more twists per day of natural (usually imported) licorice may complicate antihypertensive therapy due to enhanced sodium reabsorption and potassium excretion along with subsequent water retention.

G. Sulfites

Sulfites in food or drugs may cause severe hypersensitivity reactions in some people, particularly asthmatics.[9] Sulfiting agents have been used in foods, beverages, and pharmaceuticals as antioxidants. They include sulfur dioxide, sodium sulfite, sodium & potassium bisulfite, and sodium & potassium metabisulfite. FDA regulations require that prescription products list inactive ingredients, including sulfites. Relatively few oral or OTC drugs contain sulfites. Most wines and some beers contain sulfites, and the Bureau of Alcohol, Tobacco and Firearms plans to follow the FDA proposal to label alcoholic beverages containing 10 ppm of total sulfiting agents.[34]

H. Alcohol

Chronic alcohol intake stimulates the microsomal system responsible for the metabolism of many drugs and may cause a variety of adverse effects. Ethanol is absorbed from the alimentary canal, metabolized by the liver, and may be distributed throughout the body tissues and fluids. Absorption can be affected by the type of beverage consumed, gastrointestinal pH, alcohol concentration, and concomitant ingestion of food. Individual variation in pharmacokinetics of alcohol result from differences in hepatic function, renal function, body mass, fat and water content. Depending on the quantity of alcohol consumed and the time of ingestion, the biotransformation of some drugs can be either increased or decreased. Please see Table p. 22.

Christine H. Smith, Editor

POSSIBLE ALCOHOL-DRUG INTERACTIONS

	Drug Type	Possible Effects
††	amebacidal (Flagyl)	disulfiram-like reaction
†	analgesic (Tylenol)	↑ hepatoxicity
††	antianxiety (Equanil)	↓ sedative effect
†	anticoagulant (Coumadin)	may ↑ hypoprothrombinemic response
††	anticonvulsant (Dilantin)	↓ drug effect
††	antidepressant-tricyclic (Elavil)	↑ hepatic metabolism
††	antidepressant-MAOI (Parnate)	potentiates sedative effects
†	antifungal (Furoxone)	disulfiram-like reaction
††	antihistamine (Benadryl)	additive CNS depression
†	antineoplastic (Matulane)	disulfiram-like reaction
†	antipsychotic (Thorazine)	additive CNS depression impaired psychomotor skills
†	antitubercular (isoniazid)	↑ hepatitis, ↓ drug effect
†	anti-ulcer (Tagamet)	inhibits hepatic metabolism of alcohol
††	barbituates (Phenobarbital)	↑ hepatic alcohol metabolism
††	benzodiazepines (Valium)	impaired psychomotor skills additive CNS depression
†	beta blockers (Inderal)	↑ alcohol effects
†††	cephalosporins (Mandol, Cefobid, Moxam, Cefotan)	disulfiram reaction
†††	disulfiram (Antabuse)	rapid heart beat, chest pains, facial flushing, n&v, hypotension
†	diuretics (Lasix)	↓ blood pressure
†	insulin (various)	additive hypoglycemic effect
††	narcotic analgesic (Dilaudid)	additive CNS depression
†	NSAI (Indocin)	↑ gastric mucosal damage
†	oral hypoglycemic (Diabinese)	disulfiram-like reaction
†	salicylates (aspirin)	damage to gastric mucosa, especially in fasting state
††	sedative, hypnotic (Noctec)	impaired psychomotor skills, flushing, ↑ CNS depression

These suggestions for ETOH intake are meant as general guidelines: Consult the physician.

†   Abstinence not required, intake should be limited (1–2 oz c̄ physician's permission)

††   Abstinence recommended

††† Total abstinence required.

From: Vol 5, #4 *Drug Interactions Newsletter*, Nov. 1985; Vol 23, #7 *Medical Letter*, Apr. 1981

ALTERED NUTRITIONAL STATUS CAUSED BY ALCOHOL

Alcohol is used and abused by a large percentage of the adult populace. The recognition and correction of nutritional depletion is a major objective in the management of alcohol abuse.

ALCOHOL AND NUTRITION MAY INTERACT AT VARIOUS LEVELS

1. Displaces food from the diet:
   A. Suppresses appetite.
   B. Decreases the ingestion of essential nutrients: protein and Vit malnutrition.
2. By injuring the liver, pancreas or bowel, functions of GI tract compromised:
   A. Composition of pancreatic juice altered: may result in ductal blockage, possible maldigestion of fat and protein.
   B. Liver: Fat accumulation; protein synthesis blocked; triglyceride level increased.
   C. Stomach: Affects many facets of gastric physiology, including acid secretion, mucosal permeability, gastric emptying — may result in anorexia, abdominal pain, malnutrition.
   D. Small bowel: Direct effect is impaired absorption of fat, Vit B_6, folic acid, Vit B_{12} and Thi.
   E. Chronic alcohol abuse can enhance enzyme activity.

3. Alters metabolism and activation of dietary constituents:
   A. 1 gram of alcohol yields 7.1 kilocalories, but does not behave as other kilocaloric equivalents — oxidized differently, behaves as "empty calories."
   B. Interferes with activation of Vit B_6, Vit D metabolism may also be disturbed, contributing to increased incidence of fractures due to poor utilization of calcium.
   C. Diets deficient in both protein and kilocalories may result in muscle wasting and edema.
   D. Serum level of folic acid commonly depressed in the malnourished chronic alcoholic — may result in megaloblastic anemia.
   E. Synthesis of coagulation proteins may be abnormal due to liver injury.
   F. Possible Thi deficiency resulting in neuropathy, psychosis.
   G. Increased zinc excretion: slow wound healing.
      Increased potassium excretion: muscle weakness.
      Increased magnesium excretion: electrocardiology changes; delirium tremens.
      Possible iron overload: hemachromatosis.
   H. Brain: Impaired learning, memory.
   I. Heart disease: symptoms of cardiomyopathy — enlargement of the heart, disease of the heart muscle which was not due to disorders known to cause heart disease.
   J. Fetal Alcohol Syndrome: possible heart defects.

4. Has an immunity-weakening effect on every component of the immune system.

The degree of deficiency depends on the length of time the person has been drinking and the quality of the diet between drinking bouts. Dietary modifications may be needed to treat complications of cirrhosis, gastritis and pancreatitis. A diet rich in protein and vitamins may repair a fat-infiltrated liver. After alcohol interference of the absorptive mechanism is corrected, massive vitamin supplementation is not necessary and will not substitute for a well-balanced diet.

Before wine or any alcoholic beverage is served to patients, the physician should be consulted.

DIETARY SUGGESTIONS TO AID IN THE RELIEF OF NUTRITION RELATED SIDE EFFECTS OF DRUGS

Suggestions are intended to reinforce rather than replace any information in the diet prescription provided by the physician. It is important to keep in mind that each person is unique. Some individuals may experience only mild, transient discomforts, while others may be markedly affected by a wide spectrum of drug effects altering food intake. Prior to implementing dietary suggestions, consult physician/pharmacist to determine if the side effect is a possible adverse effect of the drug; the patient may be in need of medical attention. The following is a list of suggested changes in eating habits that may relieve unpleasant side effects of drugs:

DRUG-INDUCED SIDE EFFECT	SUGGESTIONS
Loss of Appetite	1. Question patient regarding factors contributing to appetite loss.
	2. Educate the patient to know why eating food is important.
	3. Create a pleasant environment for eating.
	4. If early satiety occurs or meals are not well-tolerated, offer small, frequent, attractive meals or snacks.
	5. Provide variety in color, texture and temperature.
	6. Enhance flavors by using various seasonings. Marinate meats in sauces or fruit juices.
	7. Encourage weakened patients to select foods that require little effort.
	8. Instruct patient to avoid excessive alcohol intake.

Taste/Smell Dysfunction

1. If permissible, advise patient to mask taste of drug with food, pulpy fruits (applesauce, crushed pineapple), fruit juices or milk.
2. Unless otherwise directed, urge patient to take medication with adequate fluid.
3. To improve taste, suggest the use of sugarless gum or water or lemon juice as mouth rinses.
4. Instruct patient to alter food types and textures.
5. Encourage good oral hygiene.

Dry or Sore Mouth

1. Counsel patient to moisten (dunk) dry foods in beverages or to swallow foods with a beverage.
2. Decrease the use of dry (or salty) foods or snacks.
3. Offer moist, soft-textured foods: mashed potatoes, pureed vegetables, milk toast without crust, custards or puddings, fruit whips, creamed ground meat or fish.
4. Avoid spicy, rough textured or highly acidic foods.
5. Add milk-flavored sauces, gravies or syrups to food.
6. Suggest that patient lick or suck on ice chips; frequent rinses with warm water may help.
7. Incorporate cold foods or beverages into meals or snacks: sherbets, ice or cold milk, ice cream, melons, fruit ices.
8. Suggest the use of sugarless gum.
9. Caution the patient that the use of hard candies may increase the incidence of dental caries.

10. Advise patient of the importance of good oral hygiene. Severe or long term decreased salivation may result in rampant tooth decay, gum disease, fungal infection, ill-fitting dentures and changes in eating habits. If dry mouth lasts 2 weeks, a dental consultation is needed.

Appetite Stimulation or Weight Gain

1. Educate patient that certain drugs may increase desire for sweets and other foods.
2. Assess weight gain as a possible reversal of depression-induced weight loss.
3. If applicable, assure the patient that after drug discontinuation (e.g., amitriptyline, a tricyclic antidepressant) that drug-related food cravings may diminish and weight may be lost.
4. Encourage intake of low-kilocaloric foods, beverages and snacks.
5. Advise patient to incorporate high fiber foods or snacks in the diet which may contribute to early satiety.
6. Instruct patient or food provider to control access to specific high kilocaloric foods, snacks, or beverages.

Epigastric Distress
(stomach discomfort, heartburn or indigestion)

1. After drug administration, particularly those medications known to cause GI irritation, suggest that patient maintain an upright posture for approximately 15 to 30 minutes.
2. Question patient about dietary habits and specific foods or beverages that may contribute to epigastric distress.
3. Offer small quantities of food at frequent intervals in a relaxed environment. Avoid overeating.

4. Instruct the patient not to homogenize, mince or puree food and to avoid extemely cold/hot foods or liquids (may stimulate acid secretion).
5. Control the use of alcohol, coffee, tea and other caffeine-containing beverages, decaffeinated coffee, cola beverages, peppermint, chocolate, pepper, and other spices or spicy food.
6. Avoid orange and other citrus juices, tomato products and other highly acidic foods, or concentrated fruit beverages if found to cause epigastric distress.
7. Advise patient to avoid greasy, fried or fatty foods (may delay gastric emptying).
8. Evaluate the intake of milk or cream (may stimulate acid secretion).
9. Urge patient to avoid eating at least one hour before bedtime.
10. If patient is overweight, advise patient to decrease food intake sensibly to lose weight.

Nausea

1. Honor the patient's food preferences.
2. Offer small quantities of easily digestible foods at frequent intervals. Instruct patient to eat slowly.
3. Reduce food volume at meals; serve liquids after meals or limit liquid intake with meals.
4. Suggest the intake of toasted or dry enriched white bread, salted or graham crackers, or cooked or dry ready-to-eat cereals. May benefit patient to ingest one of these foods early in the morning or before arising.
5. Serve cold, clear (iced tea), or carbonated (ginger ale) liquids or juices. Avoid lukewarm beverages.
6. Avoid any fried, greasy or fatty foods (may delay gastric emptying).

7. Inform the patient or food provider that hot aromas may aggravate nausea. Cold foods may be more tolerable than hot foods.
8. Reschedule meal and snack times, if nausea occurs at consistent times each day.
9. If nausea and vomiting occur, maintain adequate hydration and nutrient intake.

Diarrhea

1. Focus on fluid and electrolyte replacement.
2. During the acute phase, food may be withheld for 24 hours or longer, or the diet prescription may be restricted to clear fluids (e.g., broths, bouillon, fruit juices, ginger ale or other liquids).
3. The intake of frequent small amounts of soft foods (e.g., crackers, banana, plain toast) may be allowed as tolerated.
4. Foods that should be initially restricted or avoided include caffeine-containing foods or beverages, alcohol, candies and other concentrated sweets, raw vegetables and fruits, uncooked foods, fried foods, bran and whole grain cereals, nuts, beans, relishes and other miscellaneous foods. Milk or milk products, which are not tolerated due to decreased lactase activity, may be gradually added to the diet later.
5. If tolerated, incorporate pectin-containing foods in the diet (applesauce, grated raw apple).
6. Advise the patient to return to a normal diet gradually.

Gastrointestinal Gas
(Flatulence)

1. Educate the patient to evaluate dietary and other habits, such as eating too fast, chewing gum, and situations associated with swallowing large amounts of air.
2. Encourage patient to avoid flatulogenic foods (a matter of individual response). Some examples of gas-forming foods include beans, bran, cabbage, cauliflower, onions, pastries, radishes, apples, celery, eggplant and other foods.
3. Advise patient to limit consumption of carbonated beverages.

Constipation

1. Question patient about the prolonged use of or overuse of cathartics, laxatives, or enemas. These agents should not be used in the treatment of simple constipation as they interfere with normal bowel reflexes.
2. If applicable, educate patient concerning misconceptions about constipation.
3. Evaluate the diet for adequacy of fluid, volume, nutrients and bulk or residue (fiber).
4. Incorporate sources of bulk (vegetables, fruits, whole-grain cereals) in the diet. Bran should be used in moderation.
5. Advise patient to maintain adequate fluid or water intake.
6. Inform the patient about the importance of a daily exercise program and good health habits — regular meals and adequate diet with ample fiber, defecation reflex recognition (usually active after meals, especially breakfast), and regularity in defecation time.

GUIDELINES FOR COUNSELING MEDICATED PATIENTS

The following guidelines focus on specific information needed to educate medicated patients about potential drug-food/food-drug interactions. Some examples are given illustrating a possible diet adjustment that may be needed by patients for whom specific drugs are prescribed.
Dietitians, educate your patients! **DO THEY KNOW**:

1. **When** and **how** to take the drug?
   (Where applicable, patient may be advised to take the drug in the AM; PM; 6 hours before bedtime; on an empty stomach 1 hour before or 2 hours after meals; with food, meals or specific beverages; or at same time each day with food.)

2. Expected **side effects** and possible dietary suggestions to aid in their relief?
   (Cholestyramine treatment may cause constipation; the patient may be advised to eat adequate amounts of dietary fiber and to follow other suggestions to aid in its relief.)

3. The potential **nutritional problems** that may arise from specific medication use, especially when dietary intake is inadequate?
   (Potassium-depleting diuretics may cause hypokalemia due to an inadequate intake of high potassium-containing foods; advise patient to increase intake of foods known to be good sources of potassium.)

4. That some dietary changes or food habits (particularly after drug stabilization) may alter **drug action**?
   (A high intake of vitamin K-containing foods may impair warfarin action; evaluate dietary or food habits, then advise patient to regulate intake of foods high in vitamin K.)

5. What **foods and beverages to avoid** while taking the drug?)
   (Intake of foods high in pressor amines in patients for whom phenelzine (MAOI) is prescribed can cause a hypertensive crisis; advise patient to avoid these foods.)
6. That the concurrent intake of **alcohol** (beer, wine and other alcoholic beverages) with certain medications may modify the effects of both or may produce undesirable side effects?
   (A disulfiram-like reaction results from concurrent alcohol ingestion by patients prescribed metronidazole; advise patient to avoid alcohol.)
7. That potential interactions may occur between certain medications and **vitamin, mineral and other food supplements**?
   (Concurrent intake of calcium supplements during tetracycline administration results in impaired absorption of both; advise patient not to take supplement within 1 to 3 hours of the orally-administered drug.)
8. What **dietary modifications or restrictions** are associated with the medical condition and that such dietary changes may promote drug effectiveness?
   (Combined effects of a fat-modified diet and lovastatin therapy are additive in lowering blood cholesterol. Emphasize the importance of both dietary and drug compliance.)
9. That **drug therapy** should not be considered a substitute for dietary regulation?
   (Control of diabetes is dependent on both dietary regulation and oral hypoglycemic therapy. Emphasize the importance of both dietary and drug compliance.)
10. That their **personal dietary prescription** pertains to them, and that they should not follow dietary suggestions prescribed for others?

(Dietary restrictions for patients prescribed potassium-depleting diuretics differ for patients prescribed potassium-sparing diuretics; advise patient for whom a potassium-depleting diuretic is prescribed that drug action differs for these two medications and that serious adverse effects occur if diet prescriptions are interchanged.)

11. That they should **consult** with their dietitian or physician before modifying their diet?

12. Other pertinent information about their medications? (e.g., the **name** and **purpose** of the drug, the **duration** of therapy and that they should never take **drugs prescribed for others,** or never let others use their medications.)

Christine H. Smith, Editor

FOOD-MEDICATION INTERACTIONS

MEDICATION **CLASSIFICATION & DIETARY/RELATED SIGNIFICANCES**

Accutane ANTIACNE See *isotretinoin.*

acebutolol ANTIHYPERTENSIVE, ANTIARRHYTHMIC, beta blocker
Sectral **Drug:** May be taken s̄ regard to meals. **Diet Important:** Possible ↓ Na, ↓ cal. **GI:** Constipation, flatulence, abdominal pain. **S/Cond:** Limit alcohol. Caution c̄ diabetic: may mask signs of hypoglycemia.[13] **Other:** Weakness, headache, dizziness, **Blood/Serum:** ↑ BUN, ↓ HDL, ↑ TG, ↑ uric acid, ↑ K.[1]

acetaminophen ANALGESIC, ANTIPYRETIC
Datril **Drug:** Take c̄ food to ↓ GI distress. **GI:** No GI bleeding.
Tylenol **S/Cond:** Limit alcohol.
Blood/Serum: ↑ uric acid (false + c̄ phosphotungstate method), ↑ LDH, ↑ bilirubin.[13]

MEDICATION	CLASSIFICATION & DIETARY/RELATED SIGNIFICANCES

acetazolamide
Diamox
Parenteral: 47.13mg
Na/150mg[7]

DIURETIC, ANTIGLAUCOMA, ANTICONVULSANT
Drug: Take c̄ food 6 or more hr before bedtime. **Diet:** ↑ fluids & foods ↑ in K may be needed. **S/Cond:** Not c̄ lactation. Monitor diabetic. **Metab/Phys:** Anemias. **Other:** Anorexia, ↓ wt., n&v, diarrhea, metallic taste, lethargy.
Blood/Serum: ↓ Na, ↑ Cl, ↓ bicarbonate, ↑ bilirubin, ↑ uric acid, ↑ glucose.
Urinary: ↑ Na, ↑ K, ↓ Cl, ↑ bicarbonate, ↑ Ⓟ, ↓ citrate, ↓ uric acid, ↑ glucose, + for protein, ↑ Thi, ↑ Pyr, ↑ Ca, ↑ Mg.[11]

acetohexamide
Dymelor

ORAL HYPOGLYCEMIC
Diet Important: Take c̄ meals; not a substitute for dietary regulation. **S/Cond:** Avoid alcohol. **GI:** Diarrhea, n&v, dyspepsia, heartburn. **Metab/Phys:** Anemia. **Other:** Metallic taste.
Blood/Serum: ↓ glucose, ↓ uric acid.

acetohydroxamic acid
Lithostat

ANTI-INFECTIVE, urinary
Drug: Take 1 hr before or 2 hr after meals. **GI:** N&v. **S/Cond:** Avoid alcohol. Chelates metals, especially Fe. **Metab/Phys:** Possible hemolytic anemia. **Other:** Weakness, ↓ appetite, headache.

acetylsalicylic acid
  Aspirin
  Ecotrin
  Empirin
	ANALGESIC, NSAI, ANTIPYRETIC	

Drug: Take c̄ 8oz H$_2$O or c̄ food if GI distress. (Food ↓ absorption.) Swallow tab whole. **Diet:** May indicate need for adequate fluid intake. Need intake of foods ↑ in C & Fol. **Nutr:** lipogenesis: ↓ tryptophan.[11] − N balance. **GI:** Nausea, dyspepsia. **S/Cond:** Not for patients prone to Vit K deficiency. Limit alcohol. **Metab/Phys:** May contribute to or aggravate Fe deficiency anemia. 4–5gms/day long-term use causes 3–8ml fecal blood loss.[14]
Blood/Serum: ↓ Vit C, (rheumatoid arthritis), ↓ Fol, ↑ or ↓ uric acid, dose related, ↓ T$_4$, ↓ K.
Urinary: ↑ Vit C, ↑ K, ↑ amino acids, ↑ glucose (dose related), ↑ Thi.

Achromycin-V	ANTIBIOTIC	See ***tetracycline.***
ACTH, Acthar	CORTICOSTEROID	See ***corticotropin.***

Actifed
  triprolidine HCl
  monohydrate &
  pseudoephedrine HCl
  (plus codeine
  phosphate)
	ANTIHISTAMINIC, SYMPATHOMIMETIC, DECONGESTANT	

Drug: Take c̄ food or milk. Swallow caps whole. **GI:** Epigastric distress, n&v, diarrhea, constipation. **S/Cond:** Caution c̄ diabetic. Not c̄ lactation. **Other:** Dry mouth,[10] drowsiness, anorexia, dizziness, taste changes.[37]
Blood/Serum: ↑ amylase, ↑ lipase.

MEDICATION	CLASSIFICATION & DIETARY/RELATED SIGNIFICANCES

Actinomycin-D ANTINEOPLASTIC   See *dactinomycin.*

Acutrim APPETITE SUPPRESSANT   See *phenylpropanolamine.*

acyclovir ANTIVIRAL
   Zovirax
     Drug: Parenterally or orally administered. May take c̄ food.
     Diet: Encourage ↑ fluids unless otherwise directed. **GI:** Long term
     use: diarrhea, n&v. **Other:** Medication taste,[10] anorexia, dizziness.
     Blood/Serum: ↑ BUN, ↑ creatinine.

Adapin ANTIDEPRESSANT   See *doxepin HCl.*

Adriamycin ANTINEOPLASTIC   See *doxorubicin.*

Advil ANTI-INFLAMMATORY   See *ibuprofen.*

Agoral Plain LAXATIVE   See *mineral oil.*

albuterol sulfate BRONCHODILATOR
   Proventil
   Ventolin
     GI: N&v. **S/Cond:** Monitor diabetic:[13] ↑ blood glucose. Limit caf-
     feine. Syrup: hyperactivity in children.[3] Not c̄ lactation. **Other:** Dry
     mouth, peculiar taste, dizziness, tremor, headache.

Aldactazide	ANTIHYPERTENSIVE, DIURETIC	
	No serum Mg value. See *spironolactone* $\bar{c}$ *hydrochlorothiazide*.	
Aldactone	DIURETIC	See *spironolactone*.
Aldoclor	ANTIHYPERTENSIVE $\bar{c}$ DIURETIC	See *methyldopa*.
		See *chlorothiazide*.
Aldomet	ANTIHYPERTENSIVE	See *methyldopa*.
Aldoril	ANTIHYPERTENSIVE $\bar{c}$ DIURETIC	See *methyldopa*.
		See *hydrochlorothiazide*.
Alka-Seltzer	ANTACID	See *buffered aspirin*.
	Effervescent antacid & pain reliever $\bar{c}$ buffered aspirin — 567mg Na/tab; Alka-Seltzer effervescent antacid — 311mg Na/tab; Alka-Seltzer Plus — 506mg Na/tab; Flavored Alka-Seltzer effervescent antacid pain reliever — 506mg Na/tab.	
Alkeran	ANTINEOPLASTIC	See *melphalan*.

See "Guide to the Use of This Book" p. 5 for explanation of format.

MEDICATION	CLASSIFICATION & DIETARY/RELATED SIGNIFICANCES

allopurinol
Lopurin
Zyloprim

ANTIGOUT
> **Drug:** Take after meals c̄ fluids. **Diet:** Use 10–12 glasses fluids/day to produce 2 liters urine per 24 hr.[13] **Nutr:** ↓ risk of xanthine calculi: maintain alkaline urine. **GI:** N&v, abdominal pain. **S/Cond:** Avoid alcohol. Not c̄ Vit C supplements.[3] **Other:** Metallic taste, drowsiness.
> **Blood/Serum:** ↑ alk phos, ↑ SGOT, ↑ SGPT, ↓ uric acid.
> **Urinary:** ↓ uric acid.

alprazolam
Xanax

ANTIANXIETY, benzodiazepine
> **Drug:** Take c̄ food or H_2O to avoid GI upset. **GI:** Constipation, diarrhea, n&v. **S/Cond:** Not c̄ lactation. Avoid alcohol.
> **Other:** Drowsiness, dry mouth, blurred vision, headache, confusion, dizziness, ↑ salivation, ↑ or ↓ wt, tremors.

aluminum carbonate
Basaljel
Suspension: 2.99mg
   Na/5ml
Cap/tab: 2.76mg Na

ANTACID   See **_aluminum hydroxide._**
> **Drug:** Swallow cap whole. Take suspension in H_2O or juice.
> **Blood/Serum:** ↑ alk phos, ↓ Ⓟ (c̄ overdose).[10]

aluminum hydroxide	ANTACID
AlternaGel	**Drug:** Take 1–3 hr after meals. Chew chewables well. **Diet:** Ulcer therapy — take between meals, chew thoroughly, follow c̄ 125ml H₂O. **Diet Important:** Phosphate-binding therapy — take c̄ meals & 250ml H₂O or fluids. c̄ hyperphosphatemia: a ↓ phosphate diet may be used. **Nutr:** Inactivates Thi, ↓ absorption of Vit A & phosphate. **GI:** Constipation, cramps, bloating, n&v. **S/Cond:** Not c̄ lactation. **Metab/Phys:** Ca & Vit A deficiency: possible osteomalacia (drug induced precipitation of bile acids may ↓ Vit A absorption.)[14] **Other:** Anorexia, chalky taste.
.677gm sorbitol/5ml	
Amphojel	
2.3mg Na/5ml,	
1.81mg Na/3gm tab	
Contains sorbitol	
Alupent	BRONCHODILATOR See ***metaproterenol sulfate.***
amantadine HCl	ANTIPARKINSONISM, ANTIVIRAL
Symmetrel	**GI:** N&v, constipation,[7] **S/Cond:** Not c̄ lactation. Avoid alcohol. **Other:** Confusion, dry mouth, anorexia, blurred vision, edema. Long term: rapid ↑ wt.[13]
Syrup: 3.2gm	
sorbitol/5ml	
Amcill	ANTIBIOTIC See ***ampicillin.***

See "Guide to the Use of This Book" p. 5 for explanation of format.

MEDICATION	CLASSIFICATION & DIETARY/RELATED SIGNIFICANCES

amikacin sulfate
Amikin
29.35mg Na/gm

ANTIBIOTIC, aminoglycoside
    Drug: Parenterally administered. **Diet:** Hydration important.
    GI: N&v, stomatatis. **S/Cond:** Contains sulfites.[7] **Other:** Hearing
    loss possible.[1] Anorexia, dizziness, unusual thirst, clumsiness,
    ↑ salivation.[7]
    Blood/Serum: ↑ BUN, ↑ SGOT, ↑ SGPT, ↑ alk phos,[13] ↓ Na,
    ↑ bilirubin, ↑ creatinine, ↑ LDH, ↓ Ca, ↓ Mg, ↓ K.
    Urinary: + protein, ↓ specific gravity.[3]

amiloride HCl &
hydrochlorothiazide
Moduretic

ANTIHYPERTENSIVE, DIURETIC
    Drug: Take c̄ food at the same time each day.[7] **Diet**
    Important: ↓ Na, ↓ cal diet may be recommended. Limit
    ↑ K foods. **GI:** Nausea, diarrhea, GI pain, constipation.
    S/Cond: Monitor diabetic: possible hyperglycemia.[3] Not c̄ lactation.
    Metab/Phys: Electrolyte imbalance, anemias. **Other:** Dizziness,
    anorexia, dry mouth, headache, appetite changes.
    Blood/Serum: ↑ BUN, ↑ Ca, ↓ Ⓟ, ↓ Na, ↓ Mg, ↑ or ↓ K,
    ↓ Cl, ↑ uric acid.
    Urinary: ↓ Ca, ↓ or ↑ K, ↑ Na, ↑ Cl, ↑ uric acid.

aminocaproic acid **Amicar**	HEMOSTATIC, ANTIFIBRINOLYTIC **Drug:** Parenterally administered. **GI:** Nausea, cramps, diarrhea, stomach pain. **Other:** Dizziness, headache. **Blood/Serum:** ↑ K, especially in impaired renal function.[7]
aminophylline **Aminophyllin** **Somophyllin**	BRONCHODILATOR See listing for *theophylline.*
aminosalicylate Na **P.A.S.** **Teebacin** 154mg Na/gm[13]	ANTITUBERCULAR **Drug:** Take c̄ food or after meals. **Nutr:** ↓ B_{12} absorption.[13] **GI:** N&v, diarrhea, abdominal pain. **S/Cond:** Caution c̄ lactation. **Metab/Phys:** Blood dyscrasias. Not c̄ G6PD deficiency. **Other:** Unpleasant taste c̄ solutions. **Blood/Serum:** ↑ SGOT, ↑ SGPT. **Urinary:** ↑ glucose (possible false + c̄ $CuSO_4$).[13]
amiodarone **Cordarone**	ANTIARRYTHMIC, ANTIANGINAL **Drug:** Take c̄ food. **GI:** N&v, constipation, abdominal pain. **S/Cond:** Not c̄ lactation. **Other:** Anorexia, headache, tremor, weakness, blurred vision, abnormal taste, smell & salivation.[10] **Blood/Serum:** ↑ SGOT, ↑ SGPT, ↑ T_4, ↓ T_3,[3] ↑ creatinine, ↑ chol.

MEDICATION	CLASSIFICATION & DIETARY/RELATED SIGNIFICANCES

amitriptyline HCl
Elavil
Endep

ANTIDEPRESSANT, tricyclic
    Drug: Parenterally or orally administered. Swallow cap/tab whole. May take $\bar{c}$ food to ↓ GI distress. **Nutr:** ↑ appetite for CHO, ↑ need for Rib. **GI:** N&v, constipation, diarrhea. **S/Cond:** Avoid alcohol.[7] Limit caffeine: see Table p. 231. **Metab/Phys:** Inappropriate ADH syndrome. Blood dyscrasias.[3] **Other:** Dry mouth, altered taste, anorexia, ↑ or ↓ wt, confusion, drowsiness. **Blood/Serum:** ↑ or ↓ glucose.

amobarbital
Amytal

SEDATIVE, HYPNOTIC
    Diet: Pyridoxine: ↓ drug effects.[14] ↑ need for Fol & Vit D. **Nutr:** May ↓ Thi absorption. ↓ plasma Ca in elderly,[4] ↓ plasma Vit B_{12}. **S/Cond:** Limit alcohol. **Metab/Phys:** ↓ gastric secretion. **Other:** Dizziness, dry mouth, altered taste, drowsiness. **Urinary:** ↑ Vit C & D.

amoxapine
Asendin

ANTIDEPRESSANT, tricyclic
    Drug: Take $\bar{c}$ food, to ↓ GI upset. **Diet:** ↑ appetite for sweets. **Nutr:** ↑ need for Rib. **GI:** Constipation, flatulence, diarrhea, nausea. **S/Cond:** Avoid alcohol. Limit caffeine: see Table p. 231. **Metab/Phys:** Inappropriate ADH syndrome. Blood dyscrasias.[3]

Other: Drowsiness, dry mouth, blurred vision, altered taste, ↑ or ↓ wt.
Blood/Serum: ↑ or ↓ glucose.[13]

amoxicillin
 Amoxil
 Larotid
 Polymox
 Trimox
 Utimox
 Wymox

ANTIBIOTIC, penicillin
 Drug: May take tab & liquid form on a full or empty stomach. May be mixed c̄ formulas, milk, fruit juice, H_2O or ginger ale.[13] Chewable tabs: crush or chew. Amoxil contains sucrose.[29] **Diet:** Acid stable.[1] **GI:** N&v, diarrhea. **Metab/Phys:** Anemia.
 Blood/Serum: ↑ SGPT, ↑ SGOT.
 Urinary: False + glucose ($CuSO_4$).[13]

amoxicillin,
potassium clavulanate
 Augmentin
 "500" & "250" tabs:
  24.6mg K
 "250" powder:
  12.5mg K/5ml
  fruit flavored
 "125" powder:
  6.24mg K, fruit
  flavored for oral
  suspension[29]

ANTIBIOTIC
 Drug: May be mixed c̄ formulas, milk, fruit juice, H_2O or ginger ale. Take consistently s̄ regard to meals. **Diet:** Acid stable.
 GI: Diarrhea, n&v, gastritis. **Metab/Phys:** Anemia. **Other:** ↓ wt.
 Blood/Serum: ↑ SGOT, ↑ SGPT.
 Urinary: false + glucose ($CuSO_4$).[13]

| MEDICATION | CLASSIFICATION & DIETARY/RELATED SIGNIFICANCES |

MEDICATION

amphetamine sulfate
  Benzedrine

Amphojel

ampicillin
  Amcill
  Omnipen
  Polycillin
  Totacillin

ampicillin trihydrate
  Principen

CLASSIFICATION & DIETARY/RELATED SIGNIFICANCES

STIMULANT
  Drug: Take 6 hours or more before bedtime. Swallow extended release caps whole. **GI:** N&v, diarrhea, constipation. **Other:** Dizziness, irritability, dry mouth, anorexia, ↓ wt, metallic taste, blurred vision.[1]

ANTACID   See *aluminum hydroxide.*

ANTIBIOTIC, penicillin
  Drug: Take c̄ H_2O 1 hr before or 2 hr after meals. Amcill suspension: 1.8gm sucrose/5ml. Parenteral: 64.4mg Na/gm to 78.2mg Na/gm. **Diet:** Acid stable.[10] **GI:** Stomatitis, n&v, diarrhea. **Metab/Phys:** Possible hypokalemia,[11] anemia. **Other:** Glossitis, black, hairy tongue, taste changes.
  Blood/Serum: ↑ SGOT (especially in infants).
  Urinary: Possible false + positive glucose ($CuSO_4$).[13]

ANTIBIOTIC   See *ampicillin.*
  Suspension: 250mg Na/5ml; 3.2gm sucrose/5ml.[29]

amrinone lactate **Inocor** 0.25mg Na metabisulfate	VASODILATOR **Drug:** Parenterally administered. **Diet:** Cautiously ↑ fluids and electrolyte intake as directed.[10] **GI:** N&v, abdominal pain. **Metab/Phys:** Monitor electrolytes. **Other:** Anorexia.	
Amytal	SEDATIVE, HYPNOTIC	See ***amobarbital.***
Anacin	ANALGESIC, ANTIPYRETIC 1 tab: 400mg aspirin, 32.0mg caffeine.	See ***acetylsalicylic acid.*** See ***caffeine.***
Anaprox	ANTI-INFLAMMATORY, ANALGESIC	See ***naproxen.***
Ancef	ANTIBIOTIC	See ***cefazolin Na.***
Ancobon	ANTIFUNGAL	See ***flucytosine.***
Anspor	ANTIBIOTIC	See ***cephradine.***
Antabuse	ALCOHOL DETERRENT	See ***disulfiram.***
Antivert	ANTINAUSEANT	See ***meclizine HCl.***
Anturane	ANTIGOUT, ANTIPLATELET	See ***sulfinpyrazone.***

MEDICATION	CLASSIFICATION & DIETARY/RELATED SIGNIFICANCES	
Apresazide	ANTIHYPERTENSIVE c̄ DIURETIC	See *hydralazine HCl.* See *hydrochlorothiazide.*
Apresoline	ANTIHYPERTENSIVE	See *hydralazine HCl.*
Aquatensen methyclothiazide	DIURETIC	See listing for *hydrochlorothiazide.*
Aristocort	CORTICOSTEROID	See *triamcinolone.*
Artane	ANTIPARKINSONISM	See *trihexyphenidyl HCl.*
Asbron-G	BRONCHODILATOR, EXPECTORANT	See *theophylline.* See *guaifenesin.*
Ascriptin	ANALGESIC	See *buffered aspirin.*
Asendin	ANTIDEPRESSANT	See *amoxapine.*
Aspirin	ANALGESIC	See *acetylsalicylic acid.*
aspirin & caffeine	ANALGESIC, ANTIPYRETIC	See *acetylsalicylic acid.* See *caffeine.*

Atarax	ANTIANXIETY	See *hydroxyzine HCl*.
atenolol **Tenormin**	ANTIHYPERTENSIVE, ANTIANGINAL, beta blocker **Drug:** May take $\bar{s}$ regard to meals.[7] **GI:** Diarrhea, nausea. **S/Cond:** Caution $\bar{c}$ diabetic: may mask signs of hypoglycemia.[13] **Other:** Dizziness, drowsiness, dry mouth, mental confusion, especially in elderly, fatigue. **Blood/Serum:** ↑ TG, ↑ K, ↑ uric acid, ↓ HDL.	
atenolol & chlorothalidone **Tenoretic**	ANTIHYPERTENSIVE $\bar{c}$ DIURETIC, beta blocker **Drug:** Take on empty stomach same time each day. Swallow tabs whole. **Diet Important:** ↓ Na, ↑ K, ↓ cal diet may be needed. **GI:** Diarrhea, n&v, GI irritation, constipation. **S/Cond:** Caution $\bar{c}$ diabetic: ↑ or ↓ glucose. Not $\bar{c}$ lactation. **Metab/Phys:** Monitor fluid & electrolyte balance: possible hypokalemia, anemia.[3] **Other:** Dizziness, fatigue, drowsiness, anorexia. **Blood/Serum:** ↓ Na, ↓ K, ↑ Ca, ↓ Mg, ↓ Cl, ↓ Ⓟ, ↑ uric acid, ↑ glucose, ↑ amylase, ↑ TG, ↑ BUN, ↓ HDL.[1] **Urinary:** ↑ Na, ↑ K, ↓ Ca, ↑ Mg, ↑ Cl, ↑ bicarbonate, ↓ uric acid, ↑ glucose.	
Ativan	ANTIANXIETY	See *lorazepam*.
Atromid-S	ANTIHYPERLIPEMIC	See *clofibrate*.

See "Guide to the Use of This Book" p. 5 for explanation of format.

MEDICATION	CLASSIFICATION & DIETARY/RELATED SIGNIFICANCES
Augmentin	ANTIBIOTIC

See *amoxicillin*.
See *potassium clavulanate*.

Aventyl — ANTIDEPRESSANT — See *nortriptyline HCl*.

Azactam — ANTIBIOTIC, monobactam — See *aztreonam*.

azatadine maleate
  Optimine
ANTIHISTAMINIC, DECONGESTANT
  Drug: Take c̄ food to ↓ GI upset. **GI:** Epigastric distress,[10] n&v.[3]
  S/Cond: Avoid alcohol. **Metab/Phys:** Blood dyscrasias.
  Other: Sedation, disturbed coordination, dry mouth, anorexia,
  altered taste.

azathioprine
  Imuran
IMMUNOSUPPRESSANT, ANTIARTHRITIC
  Drug: Take c̄ food. **GI:** N&v,[13] diarrhea, stomach pain.
  S/Cond: Not c̄ lactation. **Metab/Phys:** Blood dyscrasias.
  Other: Anorexia, lethargy, sore throat, altered taste.
  Blood/Serum: ↑ SGOT, ↑ SGPT, ↑ bilirubin, ↑ alk phos, ↓ uric
  acid, ↓ albumin, ↑ amylase.
  Urinary: ↓ uric acid.

azlocillin **Azlin** 49.8mg Na/gm[7]	ANTIBIOTIC, penicillin	

Drug: Parenterally administered. **GI:** Epigastric distress, stomatitis, n&v, diarrhea, flatulence. **Other:** Disturbed taste/smell,[10] sore tongue or mouth.[13]
Blood/Serum:[10] ↓ Hb, ↓ HCT, ↑ SGOT, ↑ SGPT, ↑ LDH, ↑ alk phos, ↑ BUN, ↑ creatinine, ↓ K, ↓ uric acid, ↑ bilirubin, ↑ Na.

AzoGantanol
sulfamethoxazole & phenazopyridine
AzoGantrisin
sulfisoxazole & phenazopyridine HCl

ANTIBIOTIC, URINARY ANALGESIC

Drug: Take c̄ 8oz of H_2O on empty stomach. **Diet:** Encourage ↑ fluids unless otherwise directed. **Nutr:** May ↓ absorption of Vit K & Fol.[11] **GI:** N&v, diarrhea, abdominal pain, pancreatitis, stomatitis. **S/Cond:** Not c̄ lactation. **Metab/Phys:** Possible blood dyscrasias, edema. **Other:** Anorexia.
Blood/Serum: ↑ creatinine.
Urinary: ↑ Vit C,[11] ↑ glucose ($CuSO_4$ false +),[1] + for protein.

Azolid	NSAI	See *phenylbutazone*.
AZT	ANTIVIRAL	See *zidovudine*.

MEDICATION	CLASSIFICATION & DIETARY/RELATED SIGNIFICANCES

aztreonam
Azactam
Powder: Na-free

ANTIBIOTIC, monobactam
Drug: Parenterally administered. **GI:** Diarrhea, n&v.
S/Cond: Caution c̄ lactation. **Other:** Tinnitus, altered taste, weakness, headache, mouth ulcers.
Blood/Serum: ↑ SGOT, ↑ SGPT, ↑ alk phos, ↑ creatinine, ↑ LDH.

Azulfidine

ANTIBIOTIC   See **sulfasalazine**.

bacampicillin
Spectrobid
Suspension: 2.3gm
sucrose/5ml

ANTIBIOTIC, penicillin
Drug: Take c̄ H_2O on empty stomach.[13] **Diet:** Acid stable.[1]
GI: Stomatitis, n&v, diarrhea. **Metab/Phys:** Anemia.
Other: Glossitis, black, hairy tongue.
Blood/Serum: ↑ SGOT (especially in infants).
Urinary: ↑ K, ↑ glucose (false + c̄ $CuSO_4$).[13/10]

baclofen
Lioresal

MUSCLE RELAXANT, ANTISPASMODIC
GI: Nausea, constipation. **S/Cond:** Avoid alcohol. Monitor diabetic.
Other: Drowsiness, dizziness,[3] weakness, confusion, fatigue, altered taste, dry mouth, blurred vision.
Blood/Serum: ↑ alk phos, ↑ SGOT, ↑ glucose.

Bactocill	ANTIBIOTIC	See *oxacillin sodium*.
Bactrim	ANTIBIOTIC	See *trimethoprim c̄ sulfamethoxazole*.
Basaljel	ANTACID	See *aluminum carbonate*.
Benadryl	ANTIHISTAMINIC	See *diphenhydramine HCl*.
Benemid	ANTIGOUT	See *probenecid*.
Bentyl	ANTISPASMODIC	See *dicyclomine HCl*.
Benzedrine	STIMULANT	See *amphetamine sulfate*.

benzphetamine HCl
Didrex
25mg tabs: tartrazine

ANOREXIANT
Drug: Take last dose 6 hr before bedtime.[13] **GI:** Nausea, diarrhea, GI distress. **S/Cond:** Limit caffeine: see Table p. 231. Monitor diabetic: may ↓ glucose levels.[13] **Metab/Phys:** Possible growth suppression in children.[4] **Other:** Dizziness, dry mouth,[1] unpleasant taste.

benzquinamide HCl
Emete-con

ANTINAUSEANT
Drug: Parenterally administered. **GI:** Nausea. **Other:** Drowsiness, dry mouth, blurred vision, anorexia, tremors, ↑ salivation.

MEDICATION	CLASSIFICATION & DIETARY/RELATED SIGNIFICANCES

benztropine mesylate
Cogentin
Contains lactose

ANTIPARKINSONISM
    Drug: Take c̄ food. **GI:** Nausea, constipation. **S/Cond:** Avoid alcohol. **Other:** Dry mouth, blurred vision, ↓ appetite, mental confusion, dizziness, drowsiness.[1]

betamethasone
Celestone

CORTICOSTEROID   See listing for **hydrocortisone.**

Betapen VK

ANTIBIOTIC   See **penicillin.**

bethanechol chloride
Urecholine

CHOLINERGIC
    Drug: Take 1 hr before or 2 hr after meals.[13] **GI:** ↑ gastric motility, belching, abdominal cramps, n&v, diarrhea. **Other:** ↑ salivation. **Blood/Serum:** ↑ lipase, ↑ SGOT, ↑ amylase,[1] ↑ bilirubin.[3]

Bicillin

ANTIBIOTIC   See **penicillin.**

bisacodyl
Contains lactose,
    sucrose[10]
Dulcolax

LAXATIVE
    Drug: Take c̄ 8oz H_2O on empty stomach.[13] Swallow tabs whole. Do not take within 1 hr of eating or drinking dairy products.[13]
    Diet: High roughage diet may be recommended. **Nutr:** ↓ intestinal absorption of glucose.[11] **GI:** Abdominal cramps.
    Metab/Phys: Hypokalemia.[13]

bismuth subsalicylate **Pepto-Bismol**	ANTIDIARRHEAL, ANTINAUSEANT **S/Cond:** Monitor diabetic: possible hypoglycemia.[3] Less than 5mg Na/dose. **Metab/Phys:** Temporary darkening of stool and tongue. May produce impaction in infants and debilitated elderly. **Blood/Serum:** ↑ uric acid.[3]	
bleomycin sulfate **Blenoxane**	ANTINEOPLASTIC **Drug:** Parenterally administered. **GI:** Vomiting, stomatitis. **S/Cond:** Not c̄ lactation.[3] **Other:** Possible mouth sores/ulcers,[13] ↓ wt, taste affected,[37] ↓ appetite.	
Blocadren	ANTIHYPERTENSIVE	See *timolol maleate*.
Bonine	ANTINAUSEANT	See *meclizine HCl*.
Brethine	ANTIASTHMA	See *terbutaline sulfate*.
Bricanyl	ANTIASTHMA	See *terbutaline sulfate*.
Bristamycin	ANTIBIOTIC	See *erythromycin*.

See "Guide to the Use of This Book" p. 5 for explanation of format.

MEDICATION	CLASSIFICATION & DIETARY/RELATED SIGNIFICANCES

bromocriptine
Parlodel
Contain sulfites

ANTIPARKINSONISM, PROLACTIN INHIBITOR
Drug: Take $\bar{c}$ food to ↓ GI irritation. **GI:** N&v, abdominal cramps, constipation, diarrhea. **S/Cond:** Limit alcohol. **Other:** <u>Headache, dizziness, fatigue,</u> dry mouth, anorexia.
<u>**Blood/Serum:**</u> ↑ BUN, ↑ SGOT, ↑ SGPT, ↑ CPK, ↑ alk phos, ↑ uric acid.

Bromo-Seltzer
buffered

ANALGESIC, ANTACID   Contains 761mg Na/dose.
See listing for **acetaminophen.**

brompheniramine
maleate
Dimetane
2.42gm sugars/5ml
Dimetapp

ANTIHISTAMINIC
Drug: Take $\bar{c}$ food, milk or H_2O. Swallow tab whole. **GI:** GI distress, n&v, diarrhea, constipation. **S/Cond:** Not $\bar{c}$ lactation. <u>Avoid alcohol.</u>[13] **Other:** <u>Drowsiness,</u> dizziness, anorexia, dry mouth, altered taste,[37] <u>confusion in elderly, excitation in children.</u>

Bronkodyl

BRONCHODILATOR   See **theophylline.**

buffered aspirin
Ascriptin
325mg aspirin, 75mg
each Mg & Al
hydroxide

ANALGESIC, NSAI, ANTIPYRETIC
Drug: Take $\bar{c}$ food & 8oz H_2O.[13] **Nutr:** ↓ absorption of tryptophan.[10] **GI:** N&v, stomach pain. **S/Cond:** Limit alcohol. Caution $\bar{c}$ diabetic: large doses ↑ hypoglycemic effects.

Bufferin
324mg aspirin,
  48.6 Al glycinate &
  97.2mg Mg
  carbonate

Blood/Serum: ↑ or ↓ uric acid, dose related,[13] ↓ chol, ↓ K, ↓ T$_4$, ↓ T$_3$.[13]
Urinary: ↑ glucose ($\bar{c}$ clinitest), ↑ Vit C, ↑ amino acids, ↑ K.[11]

bumetanide
Bumex

DIURETIC
  Drug: Single dose should be taken in A.M. after breakfast. Last dose no later than 6 P.M. **Diet:** Encourage fluids unless otherwise directed. **GI:** Cramps, n&v, abdominal pain, diarrhea.
  S/Cond: Monitor diabetic: may affect glucose metabolism. Follow prescribed diet. **Metab/Phys:** Monitor electrolytes (not K-sparing).[10] May cause hypokalemia. Blood dyscrasias. **Other:** Dizziness,[10] headache, dry mouth.
  Blood/Serum: ↓ Na, ↓ Cl, ↓ Ca, ↓ K,[3] ↑ BUN, ↑ creatinine, ↑ glucose, ↑ uric acid, ↑ SGOT, ↑ SGPT.[10]
  Urinary: ↑ Na, ↑ Cl, ↑ K, ↑ Ca, ↑ glucose, ↑ Ⓟ, + protein, ↓ uric acid.

buprenorphine
Buprenex

ANALGESIC, NARCOTIC
  Drug: Parenterally administered. **GI:** N&v. **S/Cond:** Avoid alcohol.
  Other: Sedation,[10] drowsiness, dizziness, headache.
  Blood/Serum: ↑ amylase, ↑ lipase.

MEDICATION	CLASSIFICATION & DIETARY/RELATED SIGNIFICANCES

buspirone HCl
Buspar

ANTIANXIETY
> **Drug:** Take c̄ food (↑ absorption). **GI:** N&v, gastric distress, diarrhea. **S/Cond:** Avoid alcohol. **Metab/Phys:** Edema. **Other:** Dizziness, drowsiness, confusion, blurred vision, dry mouth, altered taste/smell.
> **Blood/Serum:** ↑ SGOT, ↑ SGPT.

busulfan
Myleran

ANTINEOPLASTIC
> **Diet:** Encourage ↑ fluids unless otherwise directed. **GI:** N&v, diarrhea. **Metab/Phys:** Anemias, hyperuricemia. **Other:** Glossitis, ↓ wt, dry mouth, fatigue,[10] cheilosis.

Butazolidin

NSAI   See **phenylbutazone.**

Cafergot

ANTIMIGRAINE   See **ergotamine tartrate & caffeine.**

caffeine

STIMULANT
> **Drug:** 200 mg defined as pharmacologically active dose. See Table p. 231. **Diet:** ↑ acid secretion in stomach. **GI:** Nausea, GI distress. **Metab/Phys:** May ↑ serum glucose.[1]

Calan	ANTIARRHYTHMIC, Ca-channel blocker	See ***verapamil HCl.***

calcitonin-salmon
   Calcimar

HORMONE, CALCIUM REGULATOR
   Drug: Parenterally administered. **Nutr:** Monitor OTC products ↑ in Ca & Vit D.[13] **GI:** N&v. **S/Cond:** Not c̄ lactation.
   Blood/Serum: ↓ Ca, ↓ alk phos.
   Urinary: ↑ Na, ↑ K, ↑ Mg, ↑ Cl, ↑ Ⓟ, ↑ or ↓ Ca.[3]

calcitrol
   Rocaltrol

CALCIUM REGULATOR
   Diet Important: c̄ normal renal function, adequate amounts of basic 4 food groups & fluids are needed. Supplements: not c̄ Vit D or Ca. **GI:** N&v, constipation. **Metab/Phys:** Possible ↓ growth in children. **Other:** Weakness, headache, dry mouth, metallic taste, anorexia.
   Blood/Serum: ↓ alk phos, ↑ Ca, ↑ chol, ↑ Ⓟ, ↑ Mg, ↑ BUN, ↑ SGOT, ↑ SGPT.
   Urinary: ↑ Ca, ↑ Ⓟ.

MEDICATION	CLASSIFICATION & DIETARY/RELATED SIGNIFICANCES

calcium carbonate
Tums
2.7mg Na/tab

ANTACID

Drug: Take 1–3 hr after meals. Contains 40% Ca. **Diet:** Take Fe supplements 1 or 2 hr before or after. (May ↓ Fe absorption.) As an antacid, do not take c̄ large amounts of dairy products. Ca supplements: do not take c̄ bran, whole grain cereals, or foods ↑ in oxalates.[13] Vitamin D, concurrent use and long term therapy may result in milk-alkali syndrome. Fe, insoluble complexes may form c̄ long term use.[14] **Nutr:** Infrequent hypercalcemia c̄ alkalosis. **GI:** Belching, nausea, constipation, steatorrhea. **Other:** Chalky taste.

calcium gluconate

ANTACID Contains 9% Ca.

calcium lactate

ANTACID Contains 13% Ca.[4]

captopril
Capoten

ANTIHYPERTENSIVE

Drug: Take on empty stomach, 1 hr before meals. **Diet Important:** ↓ Na, ↓ cal, diet may be recommended. Monitor salt substitutes & K supplements. **S/Cond:** Caution c̄ lactation. **Metab/Phys:** Monitor electrolytes. Hyperkalemia. Anemias. **Other:** Altered taste,[10] ↓ wt, dizziness, sore mouth. **Blood/Serum:** ↑ BUN, ↑ creatinine, ↑ K, ↓ Na. **Urinary:** ↑ acetone (test interference[3]), + protein.

Carafate	ANTIULCER	See *sucralfate*.
carbamazepine **Tegretol**	ANTICONVULSANT **Drug:** Take c̄ food.[13] **GI:** N&v, constipation. **S/Cond:** Not c̄ lactation. Monitor diabetic. **Metab/Phys:** Blood dyscrasias, hyponatremia. Inappropriate ADH syndrome. **Other:** Dizziness, drowsiness, dry mouth, blurred vision, anorexia, altered taste.[29] **Blood/Serum:** ↑ BUN,[3] ↑ SGOT, ↑ SGPT, ↑ bilirubin, ↓ Ca, ↓ T_3, ↓ T_4. **Urinary:** ↑ glucose, albumin.	
carbenicillin disodium **Geopen** **Pyopen**	ANTIBIOTIC, penicillin See listing for *carbenicillin indanyl Na.* **Drug:** Parenterally administered. 108–150mg Na/gm. **S/Cond:** Not c̄ ↓ Na diet. Acid labile.	
carbenicillin indanyl sodium **Geocillin** Acid stable[4] 23mg Na/tab	ANTIBIOTIC, penicillin **Drug:** Take c̄ 8oz H_2O on empty stomach.[13] **GI:** N&v, stomatitis, diarrhea, flatulence. **Metab/Phys:** Monitor electrolytes: possible hypokalemia.[4] Anemia. **Other:** furry tongue, bitter taste. **Blood/Serum:** ↑ SGOT, ↑ SGPT.	
Cardarone	ANTIARRHYTHMIC	See *aminodarone.*
Cardizem	ANTIANGINAL, Ca-channel blocker	See *diltiazem HCl.*

MEDICATION	CLASSIFICATION & DIETARY/RELATED SIGNIFICANCES

carisoprodol
  Rela
  Soma

MUSCLE RELAXANT
  Drug: Contains 200mg carisoprodol & 325mg aspirin. **GI:** N&v, epigastric distress. **S/Cond:** Avoid alcohol. Not c̄ lactation. **Other:** <u>Drowsiness</u>, dizziness, confusion, tremors, visual problems, hiccups.

Castor Oil
  ricinus communis

CATHARTIC
  Drug: Take in juice or carbonated beverages on empty stomach. **Diet:** Encourage ↑ fluids unless otherwise directed. **Nutr:** ↓ absorption of Vit A, E, D & K. **Metab/Phys:** Electrolyte imbalance. **Other:** Dehydration.

Catapres

ANTIHYPERTENSIVE   See *clonidine HCl.*

Ceclor

ANTIBIOTIC   See *cefaclor.*

CeeNU

ANTINEOPLASTIC   See *lomustine.*

cefaclor
  Ceclor
  3.0gm sucrose/5ml

ANTIBIOTIC, cephalosporin
  Drug: Take s̄ regard to meals. **Diet:** Acid stable. **Nutr:** ↓ Vit K. **GI:** <u>Diarrhea</u>, n&v, stomach cramps. **S/Cond:** Caution c̄ lactation. **Metab/Phys:** Hypokalemia, hemolytic anemia. **Other:** Sore mouth

&tongue.
Blood/Serum: ↑ alk phos, ↑ SGOT, ↑ SGPT, ↑ BUN, ↑ creatinine.
Urinary: ↑ glucose (false + $\bar{c}$ CuSO$_4$).

cefadroxil
Duricef
Ultracef

ANTIBIOTIC   See listing for *cephalexin.*

Cefadyl

ANTIBIOTIC   See *cephapirin sodium.*

cefamandole nafate
Mandol
77mg Na/gm

ANTIBIOTIC, cephalosporin
Drug: Parenterally administered. **GI:** N&v, diarrhea. **S/Cond:** Avoid alcohol: Disulfiram-like reaction. **Metab/Phys:** ↓ bacterial synthesis of Vit K in intestines. **Other:** Altered taste.[3]
Blood/Serum: ↑ SGOT, ↑ SGPT, ↑ alk phos, ↑ BUN, ↑ creatinine.
Urinary: ↑ glucose (false + $\bar{c}$ CuSO$_4$), ↑ creatinine.

cefazolin sodium
Ancef
46mg Na/vial
Kefzol
48.3mg Na/gm[7]

ANTIBIOTIC, cephalosporin
Drug: Parenterally administered. **GI:** Diarrhea, stomach cramps.
Other: Sore mouth, ↓ wt.
Blood/Serum: ↑ SGOT, ↑ SGPT, ↑ alk phos, ↑ BUN.[13]
Urinary: ↑ glucose (false + $\bar{c}$ CuSO$_4$).

64

MEDICATION	CLASSIFICATION & DIETARY/RELATED SIGNIFICANCES

Cefizox ANTIBIOTIC See *ceftizoxime sodium.*

Cefobid ANTIBIOTIC See *cefoperazone.*

cefonicid sodium
 Monocid
 85mg Na/gm powder

ANTIBIOTIC, cephalosporin
 Drug: Parenterally administered. **GI:** Diarrhea.
 Blood/Serum: ↑ SGOT, ↑ SGPT, ↑ LDH, ↑ alk phos.[13]

cefoperazone
 Cefobid
 34.5mg Na/gm

ANTIBIOTIC, cephalosporin
 Drug: Parenterally administered. **GI:** Diarrhea,[4] cramps.
 S/Cond: Avoid alcohol: Disulfiram-like reaction.[9]
 Metab/Phys: ↓ bacterial synthesis of Vit K in intestines.
 Blood/Serum: ↑ alk phos, ↑ SGOT, ↑ SGPT, ↑ BUN, ↑ creatinine, ↓ HCT or ↓ Hb.[10]
 Urinary: ↑ glucose (false + $\bar{c}$ $CuSO_4$).

ceforanide
 Precef
 Powder contains
  no Na

ANTIBIOTIC, cephalosporin
 Drug: Parenterally administered. **GI:** N&v, diarrhea. **Other:** Headache, confusion.[10]
 Blood/Serum: ↑ alk phos, ↑ SGOT, ↑ SGPT, ↑ creatinine, ↑ BUN.

cefotaxime sodium
Claforan
50.6mg Na/gm

ANTIBIOTIC, cephalosporin
    Drug: Parenterally administered. **GI:** Colitis, diarrhea.
    Other: Headache.
    Blood/Serum: ↑ BUN, ↑ alk phos, ↑ SGOT, ↑ SGPT, ↑ LDH.

cefotetan disodium
Cefotan
80mg Na/gm

ANTIBIOTIC, cephalosporin   See listing for ***cefamandole nafate.***

cefoxitin
Mefoxin
54mg Na/gm

ANTIBIOTIC, cephalosporin
    Drug: Parenterally administered. **Metab/Phys:** Anemias.
    Blood/Serum: ↑ BUN, ↑ SGOT, ↑ SGPT, ↑ LDH, ↑ alk phos.
    Urinary: ↑ glucose (false + $\bar{c}$ $CuSO_4$).

ceftazidime
Fortaz
54mg Na/gm,
  contains dextrose
Tazidime
52mg Na/gm

ANTIBIOTIC, cephalosporin
    Drug: Parenterally administered. **GI:** Diarrhea. **Other:** Headache, dizziness.
    Blood/Serum: ↑ SGOT, ↑ SGPT, ↑ LDH, ↑ BUN, ↑ alk phos.

| MEDICATION | CLASSIFICATION & DIETARY/RELATED SIGNIFICANCES |

MEDICATION

ceftizoxime sodium
Cefizox
59.8mg Na/gm

ANTIBIOTIC, cephalosporin
    Drug: Parenterally administered. **GI:** Diarrhea, n&v.
    Metab/Phys: Anemias.
    Blood/Serum: ↑ alk phos, ↑ SGOT, ↑ SGPT, ↑ BUN, ↑ bilirubin, ↑ creatinine.

ceftriaxone sodium
Rocephin
83mg Na/gm

ANTIBIOTIC, cephalosporin
    Drug: Parenterally administered. **Diet:** Possible Vit K deficiency.
    GI: Diarrhea, n&v, flatulence. **S/Cond:** Caution c̄ lactation.
    Other: Altered taste, headache, dizziness, sore mouth.
    Blood/Serum: ↑ BUN, ↑ creatinine, ↑ SGPT, ↑ SGOT, ↑ alk phos, ↑ bilirubin.
    Urinary: ↑ glucose (false + c̄ $CuSO_4$).

cefuroxime sodium
Zinacef
54.2mg Na/gm
5% dextrose

ANTIBIOTIC, cephalosporin
    Drug: Parenterally administered. **GI:** Diarrhea, stomatitis.
    Metab/Phys: Blood dyscrasias.
    Blood/Serum: ↑ BUN, ↑ creatinine, ↑ SGOT, ↑ SGPT, ↑ LDH, ↑ alk phos, ↑ bilirubin, ↓ Hb, ↓ HCT.[10]

Celestone
betamethasone

CORTICOSTEROID
    Syrup: 1% alcohol, sorbitol/120ml.
    See listing for **hydrocortisone**.

Centrax	ANTIANXIETY	See ***prazepam.***

cephalexin
Keflex
Caps: no Na

ANTIBIOTIC, cephalosporin
    Drug: May take c̄ food or milk. **Diet:** Acid stable. **GI:** Diarrhea, dyspepsia. **Metab/Phys:** May ↓ synthesis of Vit K. **Other:** Dizziness, ↓ wt, sore mouth,[13] headache.
    Blood/Serum: ↑ alk phos, ↑ SGOT, ↑ SGPT.
    Urinary: ↑ glucose (false + c̄ $CuSO_4$).

cephalothin sodium
Keflin
99mg Na/gm

ANTIBIOTIC, cephalosporin
    Drug: Parenterally administered. **Nutr:** May ↓ absorption of Vit K. **GI:** Diarrhea. **Metab/Phys:** Anemia. **Other:** Sore mouth.
    Blood/Serum: ↑ alk phos, ↑ BUN, ↑ SGOT, ↑ SGPT.
    Urinary: ↑ glucose (false + c̄ $CuSO_4$).

cephapirin sodium
Cefadyl
54mg Na/gm

ANTIBIOTIC, cephalosporin
    Drug: Parenterally administered. **GI:** Diarrhea, n&v.
    Metab/Phys: ↓ bacterial synthesis of Vit K in intestines,[16] hypokalemia, hemolytic anemia. **Other:** Sore mouth & tongue.
    Blood/Serum: ↑ alk phos, ↑ SGOT, ↑ SGPT, ↑ BUN, ↑ bilirubin.
    Urinary: ↑ glucose (false + c̄ $CuSO_4$).

MEDICATION	CLASSIFICATION & DIETARY/RELATED SIGNIFICANCES

cephradine
  Anspor
    Cap: lactose/sucrose
      & no Na
  Velosef
    IV: 136mg Na/gm[7]

ANTIBIOTIC, cephalosporin
  Drug: If GI distress, take $\bar{c}$ food or milk. **Diet:** Acid stable.[10]
  GI: Diarrhea. **Other:** Sore mouth.
  Blood/Serum: ↑ SGOT, ↑ SGPT, ↑ alk phos.
  Urinary: ↑ glucose (false + $\bar{c}$ $CuSO_4$).

Cephulac　　　　　ANTIHYPERAMMONEMIC　　　　　See **lactulose.**

Cerubidine　　　　ANTINEOPLASTIC　　　　　　　　See **daunorubicin HCl.**

chenodiol
  Chenix

GALLSTONE-DISSOLUTION
  Drug: Take $\bar{c}$ food or milk. **Diet:** ↑ fiber, ↓ fat, wt controlled.
  GI: Diarrhea, cramps, n&v , flatulence, stomach pain, constipation,
  heartburn. **S/Cond:** Not $\bar{c}$ lactation. Monitor serum cholesterol.
  Other: Anorexia.
  Blood/Serum: ↑ SGPT, ↑ or ↓ uric acid (dose-related), ↑ LDL,
  ↑ SGOT, ↓ TG (women), ↑ chol.

chloral hydrate
Noctec
Syrup: 9% sucrose
Elixir: 4mg Na/10ml
0.13mg K/10ml

SEDATIVE, HYPNOTIC
Drug: Take c̄ 8oz chilled liquid to mask taste.[1] Swallow capsule whole. **GI:** Epigastric distress, n&v, flatulence, diarrhea. **S/Cond:** Avoid alcohol. **Other:** Unpleasant taste, drowsiness.
Urinary: ↑ glucose ($CuSO_4$).

chlorambucil
Leukeran

ANTINEOPLASTIC
Drug: Take c̄ chilled liquid. **Diet:** Encourage ↑ fluids unless otherwise directed. Avoid acidic foods, hot foods and spices. **GI:** N&v, GI pain. **S/Cond:** Not c̄ lactation. **Metab/Phys:** Leukemia. **Other:** Mouth sores/ulcers, sore throat, metallic taste.
Blood/Serum: ↑ uric acid.[3]
Urinary: ↑ uric acid.[3]

chloramphenicol
Chloromycetin
52mg Na/1gm vial
Suspension: 1.5gm
sucrose/5ml[29]

ANTIBIOTIC
Drug: Take c̄ 8oz of H_2O on empty stomach. Take drug 1 hr before or 2 hr after meals. **Nutr:** May ↑ need for Rib, Pyr, & Vit B_{12}. **GI:** N&v, diarrhea. **S/Cond:** Not c̄ lactation. **Metab/Phys:** Blood dyscrasias, anemia. **Other:** Bad taste, glossitis, confusion, blurred vision.
Urinary: ↑ glucose (false + c̄ $CuSO_4$).

MEDICATION	CLASSIFICATION & DIETARY/RELATED SIGNIFICANCES

chlordiazepoxide
Libritabs
Librium

ANTIANXIETY, benzodiazepine
Drug: Swallow extended release caps whole. **GI:** N&v, constipation. **S/Cond:** Limit alcohol. **Metab/Phys:** Edema, blood dyscrasias. **Other:** Dizziness, drowsiness.

Chloromycetin

ANTIBIOTIC   See *chloramphenicol.*

chlorothiazide
Diuril
500mg Na/20ml vial

ANTIHYPERTENSIVE, DIURETIC
Drug: Take c̄ food 6 or more hr before bedtime. **Diet:** Avoid natural licorice. **Diet Important:** May need a ↓ Na, ↑ K diet. ↑ need for foods high in Zn, Mg, Rib. Supplements: Caution c̄ Vit D or Ca. **Nutr:** Long term use: ↑ bone Ca. **GI:** N&v, diarrhea, constipation. **S/Cond:** Not c̄ lactation. Limit alcohol. Monitor diabetic.[1]
Metab/Phys: Monitor electrolytes. Blood dyscrasias.
Other: Anorexia, dizziness, dry mouth.
Blood/Serum: ↑ uric acid, ↑ Ca, ↓ Na, ↓ K,[10] ↓ Cl, ↓ bicarbonate, ↓ Ⓟ, ↓ Mg, ↑ or ↓ glucose.[3]
Urinary: ↑ Na, ↑ K,[3] ↑ Cl, ↑ bicarbonate, ↑ uric acid, ↑ Rib, ↑ Thi, ↑ Mg, ↑ Zn, ↓ Ca.[7]

chlorpheniramine **Teldrin**	ANTIHISTAMINIC, DECONGESTANT **Drug:** Take $\bar{c}$ food or H_2O. Do not crush tab. **GI:** N&v, GI distress, constipation. **S/Cond:** Limit alcohol. **Metab/Phys:** Anemia. **Other:** Drowsiness, dizziness, dry mouth, anorexia.
chlorpromazine HCl **Thorazine** Vials & ampules: contain sulfites[7]	ANTIPSYCHOTIC **Drug:** Take $\bar{c}$ food or H_2O. Swallow spansules whole. **Diet:** ↑ need for Rib. **Nutr:** Interferes $\bar{c}$ Rib metabolism.[11] May ↓ absorption of Vit B_{12}. **GI:** Constipation. **S/Cond:** Monitor diabetic: hyperglycemia or hypoglycemia. **Metab/Phys:** Blood dyscrasias, edema. **Other:** Dizziness, dry mouth, drowsiness, tremor, blurred vision, ↑ appetite, ↑ wt. **Blood/Serum:** ↑ chol, ↑ bilirubin (false elevation).
chlorpropamide **Diabinese**	ORAL HYPOGLYCEMIC **Drug:** Usually given at breakfast. **Diet:** Prescribed diet compliance important. **GI:** Dyspepsia, n&v. **S/Cond:** Avoid alcohol. **Metab/Phys:** Possible disulfiram-like reaction & Inappropriate ADH syndrome. Edema. **Other:** Dizziness, metallic taste, anorexia. **Blood/Serum:** ↑ alk phos, ↓ glucose, ↓ Na. **Urinary:** ↓ glucose.

See "Guide to the Use of This Book" p. 5 for explanation of format.

| MEDICATION | CLASSIFICATION & DIETARY/RELATED SIGNIFICANCES |

MEDICATION

CLASSIFICATION & DIETARY/RELATED SIGNIFICANCES

chlorthalidone
Hygroton

ANTIHYPERTENSIVE, DIURETIC

 Drug: Take c̄ food 6 or more hr before bedtime. **Diet Important:** May need a ↓ Na, ↑ K, ↑ Mg, ↑ Rib diet. Avoid natural licorice. **Nutr:** Long term use: ↓ CHO tolerance. **GI:** GI irritation, n&v, diarrhea, constipation. **S/Cond:** Not c̄ lactation. Limit alcohol. Monitor diabetic. **Metab/Phys:** Monitor electrolytes. Blood dyscrasias. **Other:** Anorexia, dizziness, dry mouth.
 Blood/Serum: ↑ uric acid, ↑ Ca, ↓ Na, ↓ K, ↓ Cl, ↓ bicarbonate, ↓ ℗, ↓ Mg, ↑ or ↓ glucose, ↑ chol, ↑ TG, ↑ LDL.
 Urinary: ↑ Na, ↑ K,[10] ↑ Cl, ↑ bicarbonate, ↑ uric acid, ↑ Rib, ↑ Thi, ↑ Mg, ↑ Pyr, ↑ Ca,[11] ↑ glucose.

chlorzoxazone
Paraflex

MUSCLE RELAXANT, ANALGESIC

 Drug: Take c̄ food or H_2O. **GI:** GI distress, constipation, n&v. **S/Cond:** Not c̄ lactation. Limit alcohol. **Metab/Phys:** Jaundice. **Other:** Drowsiness, dizziness.

Choledyl

BRONCHODILATOR   See *oxtriphylline.*

cholestyramine
Questran
Contains
  tartrazine,
  3.79gm sucrose/
  9gm packet
	ANTIHYPERLIPEMIC
	Drug: Take $\bar{c}$ H$_2$O or pureed foods; never take dry or $\bar{c}$ carbonated beverages.[13] **Diet Important:** fat modified, ↓ chol, ↑ fluids, ↑ fiber. **Nutr:** May ↓ absorption of Ca, fat, Vit A, D, K, B$_{12}$, Fol, MCT, & glucose.[11] ↓ Fe reserves: long term use. **GI:** <u>Constipation</u>, nausea, <u>flatulence</u>, indigestion, steatorrhea. **Metab/Phys:** Monitor TG & chol. Edema, osteomalacia, hyperchloremic acidosis. **Other:** Anorexia, ↑ or ↓ wt, altered taste acuity.
	Blood/Serum: ↑ TG, ↓ chol, ↓ LDL,[10] ↓ Ca, ↓ K, ↓ Na, ↑ alk phos, ↑ SGOT, ↑ SGPT, ↑ P, ↑ Cl.	

Choloxin	ANTIHYPERLIPEMIC	See *dextrothyroxine*.
Chronulac	LAXATIVE	See *lactulose*.
Chrystodigin	CARDIOTONIC	See *digitoxin*.
cimetidine **Tagamet**	ANTISECRETORY, ANTIULCER **Drug:** Take $\bar{c}$ food. **GI:** ↓ gastric secretion, diarrhea. **S/Cond:** Not $\bar{c}$ lactation. Limit caffeine. See Table p. 231. **Metab/Phys:** Monitor those predisposed to hyperglycemia. **Other:** Dizziness, confusion, especially in elderly. **Blood/Serum:** ↑ creatinine, ↑ SGOT, ↑ SGPT.	

See "Guide to the Use of This Book" p. 5 for explanation of format.

74

MEDICATION	CLASSIFICATION & DIETARY/RELATED SIGNIFICANCES

cinoxacin
Cinobac

ANTI-INFECTIVE, urinary
   Drug: Take c̄ food at same time each day. **GI:** N&v, cramps, diarrhea. **S/Cond:** Not c̄ lactation. **Metab/Phys:** Edema.[3]
   Other: Headache, dizziness, anorexia.
   Blood/Serum: ↑ BUN, ↑ SGOT, ↑ SGPT, ↑ creatinine, ↑ alk phos.

ciproxfloxacin
Cipro

ANTI-INFECTIVE, fluoroquinolone
   Drug: Take s̄ regard to meals. **GI:** N&v, diarrhea, abdominal pain. **S/Cond:** Not c̄ lactation. Caution c̄ caffeine-containing beverages; see Table p. 231. **Other:** Headache, dizziness, confusion, blurred vision.[9]
   Blood/Serum: ↑ SGOT, ↑ SGPT, ↑ alk phos, ↑ LDH, ↑ bilirubin, ↑ creatinine, ↑ BUN.[7]

cisplatin
Platinol

ANTINEOPLASTIC
   Drug: Parenterally administered. **Diet:** Encourage ↑ fluids unless otherwise directed. **GI:** N&v. **S/Cond:** Not c̄ lactation.
   Metab/Phys: Peripheral edema. **Other:** Altered taste, fatigue.
   Blood/Serum: ↑ BUN, ↑ uric acid, ↑ SGOT, ↑ SGPT, ↓ Mg, ↓ Ca, ↓ K, ↓ ℗, ↑ creatinine.

Claforan	ANTIBIOTIC	See *cefotaxime sodium.*

clindamycin HCl   ANTIBIOTIC
  Cleocin
  Contains tartrazine
  Solution: 1.5gm
    sucrose/5ml

    Drug: May take c̄ meals or 8oz H_2O. **GI:** Severe colitis, n&v, flatulence, diarrhea, cramps. **S/Cond:** Not c̄ lactation.
    Metab/Phys: Hypokalemia. **Other:** Bitter taste, bloating, anorexia, ↓ wt, ↑ thirst.
    Blood/Serum: ↑ alk phos, ↑ SGOT, ↑ SGPT.

Clinoril	NSAI	See *sulindac.*

clofibrate   ANTIHYPERLIPEMIC
  Atromid-S

    Drug: Take c̄ meals. **Diet:** Diet ↓ in fat, sugar, & chol recommended.[13] **Nutr:** ↓ absorption of carotene, glucose, Fe, MCT, Vit B_{12}, electrolytes. **GI:** Nausea, diarrhea, flatulence, GI distress.
    Metab/Phys: Anemias.[11] **Other:** Aftertaste, altered taste,[37] ↑ appetite, weakness.
    Blood/Serum: ↑ SGOT, ↑ SGPT, ↑ CPK.
    Urinary: + protein.

MEDICATION	CLASSIFICATION & DIETARY/RELATED SIGNIFICANCES
clonazepam **Klonopin**	ANTICONVULSANT, benzodiazepine **GI:** Constipation, diarrhea, nausea. **S/Cond:** Not c̄ lactation. Avoid alcohol. **Metab/Phys:** Anemia. **Other:** Drowsiness, clumsiness, anorexia, coated tongue, dry/sore mouth, appetite, ↑ or ↓. **Blood/Serum:** ↑ SGOT, ↑ SGPT, ↑ alk phos.
clonidine HCl **Catapres**	ANTIHYPERTENSIVE **Diet Important:** ↓ Na diet and/or ↓ cal may be recommended. **GI:** N&v, constipation. **S/Cond:** Limit alcohol. **Metab/Phys:** Edema. **Other:** Dry mouth, drowsiness, dizziness, ↑ wt. **Blood/Serum:** ↑ glucose, ↑ CPK. **Urinary:** ↑ aldosterone.
clorazepate dipotassium **Tranxene**	ANTIANXIETY, ANTICONVULSANT, benzodiazepine **GI:** Constipation. **S/Cond:** Not c̄ lactation. Avoid alcohol. **Metab/Phys:** Edema. **Other:** Drowsiness, dizziness, dry mouth, confusion, hiccups, blurred vision.
clotrimazole **Mycelex (Troche)**	ANTIFUNGAL **Drug:** Do not chew or swallow lozenge whole.[7] Dissolve slowly in mouth. Swallow saliva. **GI:** N&v. **Blood/Serum:** ↑ SGOT.

cloxacillin sodium **Cloxapen** 13.2–15mg Na/250 tab **Tegopen** Contains no Na	ANTIBIOTIC, penicillin **Drug:** Take c̄ 8oz of H_2O on empty stomach. **Diet:** Acid stable. **GI:** Nausea, epigastric distress, diarrhea. **S/Cond:** Not c̄ lactation. **Blood/Serum:** ↑ SGOT.	
codeine	ANTITUSSIVE, ANALGESIC, NARCOTIC **Drug:** Take c̄ food or H_2O to ↓ n&v. **GI:** N&v. To avoid constipation ↑ fluids, ↑ fiber. **S/Cond:** Avoid alcohol. **Other:** Anorexia, drowsiness.	
Cogentin	ANTIPARKINSONISM	See ***benztropine mesylate.***
Colace	STOOL SOFTENER	See ***docusate sodium.***
ColBenemid	ANTIGOUT	See ***probenecid*** & ***colchicine.***

MEDICATION	CLASSIFICATION & DIETARY/RELATED SIGNIFICANCES

colchicine
Colchicine

ANTIGOUT

    Drug: Take c̄ H_2O. Use 10–12 glasses fluid/day. **Diet:** During acute attack, may need ↓ purine diet. **Nutr:** Cobalamin: absorption may be ↓ due to drug-induced functional changes in the ileal mucosa.[7] May ↓ absorption of Vit A, Fol, K, fat, Na, N, lactose.[11] **GI:** Abdominal pain,[1] n&v, diarrhea. **S/Cond:** Limit alcohol. Gradual wt loss may be suggested. **Metab/Phys:** Blood dyscrasias. **Other:** Burning throat, ↓ appetite, altered taste.[37] **Blood/Serum:** ↓ chol, ↓ Vit A, ↓ B_{12},[11] ↑ alk phos, ↑ SGOT.[13]

colestipol
Colestid

ANTIHYPERLIPEMIC

Contains no sucrose or tartrazine.
See listing for *cholestyramine.*

Combipres

ANTIHYPERTENSIVE, DIURETIC

See *chlorthalidone.*
See *clonidine HCl.*

Compazine

ANTIPSYCHOTIC

See *prochlorperazine.*

Control

APPETITE SUPPRESSANT

See *phenylpropanolamine.*

Corgard

ANTIHYPERTENSIVE, ANTIANGINAL

See *nadolol.*

Correctol

CATHARTIC

See *phenolphthalein.*

Cortef	CORTICOSTEROID	See *hydrocortisone*.
corticotropin (IV) ACTH Acthar	CORTICOSTEROID **Drug:** Take c̄ food to ↓ GI distress. **Diet Important:** Limit Na. ↑ need of protein, Ca, Vit D, Vit C, Fol,[1] Pyr, K.[11] **Nutr:** ↓ absorption of Ca,[29] P, − N balance. **GI:** Esophagitis. **S/Cond:** Monitor diabetic: prolonged use will ↓ CHO metabolism & change lipid metabolism. Not c̄ lactation. **Metab-/Phys:** Electrolyte imbalance. Pacreatitis. **Other:** Bloating, blurred vision, ↑ appetite, ↑ wt (Na retention). **Blood/Serum:** ↑ glucose, ↑ TG, ↑ chol, ↓ Zn.[11]	
Cortisol	CORTICOSTEROID	See *hydrocortisone*.
Cosmegen	ANTINEOPLASTIC	See *dactinomycin*.
Coumadin	ANTICOAGULANT	See *warfarin sodium*.
cromolyn sodium Intal Cap: 20mg lactose	ANTIASTHMA **Other:** Dizziness, headache, dry throat, bad taste.[11]	
Crystodigin	CARDIOTONIC	See *digitoxin*.
Cuprimine	METAL CHELATING AGENT	See *penicillamine*.

MEDICATION	CLASSIFICATION & DIETARY/RELATED SIGNIFICANCES

cyclobenzaprine
Flexeril

MUSCLE RELAXANT
    GI: Nausea, constipation. **S/Cond:** Not c̄ lactation. Avoid alcohol.
    Other: Drowsiness, dizziness, dry mouth, unpleasant taste,
    tremors, blurred vision.

Cyclopar

ANTIBIOTIC   See ***tetracycline.***

cyclophosphamide
Cytoxan

ANTINEOPLASTIC
    Drug: Take tabs during or after meals. **Diet:** Encourage ↑ fluids
    unless otherwise directed. **GI:** N&v. **Metab/Phys:** Inappropriate
    ADH syndrome. Anemia. **Other:** Anorexia, mucosal ulceration,
    weakness.
    Blood/Serum: ↑ uric acid.
    Urinary: ↑ uric acid.

cycloserine
Seromycin

ANTIBIOTIC, ANTITUBERCULAR
    Drug: Take c̄ food. **Diet:** ↑ need of Fol, Pyr, Vit B$_{12}$.
    Nutr: ↓ absorption of Ca, Mg. **S/Cond:** Not c̄ lactation. Avoid
    alcohol. **Other:** Drowsiness, dizziness, confusion, headache.
    Blood/Serum: ↑ SGOT, ↑ SGPT.

cyclosporine **Sandimmune**	IMMUNOSUPPRESSANT	

Drug: Oral solution: Mix at room temperature & dilute c̄ milk, chocolate milk or orange juice.[7] Take at same time each day.
GI: N&v, diarrhea. **Metab/Phys:** Anemia, hyperglycemia.
Other: Gum inflammation, tremors, headache, anorexia.
Blood/Serum: ↑ SGPT, ↑ alk phos, ↑ SGOT, ↑ bilirubin, ↑ amylase, ↑ K, ↑ uric acid, ↓ Mg, ↑ K.

cyprohepatadine HCl
Periactin
Syrup: 5% alcohol — ANTIHISTAMINIC, ANTIPURITIC

Drug: Take c̄ food, H$_2$O or milk. **GI:** Constipation, n&v.
S/Cond: Not c̄ lactation. Avoid alcohol. May be used as an appetite stimulant. **Metab/Phys:** Edema, blood dyscrasias.[10]
Other: Drowsiness, dry mouth, ↑ wt, ↑ appetite, blurred vision, altered taste, confusion, tremors.

Cytomel	THYROID HORMONE	See *liothyronine sodium.*
Cytoxan	ANTINEOPLASTIC	See *cyclophosphamide.*

MEDICATION	CLASSIFICATION & DIETARY/RELATED SIGNIFICANCES

dactinomycin
 Actinomycin-D
 Cosmegen

ANTINEOPLASTIC
   Drug: Parenterally administered. **Diet:** Encourage ↑ fluids unless otherwise directed. For children in radiation therapy, use gluten & lactose-free diet. ↑ need of Vit B_{12}, & snacks of ↑ nutrient density.[29] **Nutr:** ↓ absorption of Ca, Fe, fat.[11] **GI:** N&v, diarrhea, heartburn. **Metab/Phys:** Anemia. **Other:** Anorexia, oral ulcerations, fatigue.
   Blood/Serum: ↑ uric acid.
   Urinary: ↑ uric acid.

Dalmane

HYPNOTIC   See **flurazepam HCl.**

dantrolene sodium
 Dantrium

MUSCLE RELAXANT
   GI: Diarrhea,[1] gastric bleeding. **S/Cond:** Not c̄ lactation. Avoid alcohol. **Other:** Drowsiness, dizziness, fatigue, altered taste, anorexia.
   Blood/Serum: ↑ alk phos, ↑ SGOT, ↑ SGPT, ↑ bilirubin.

Darvocet-N

ANALGESIC   See listing for **propoxyphene HCl.**

Darvon **Darvon Compound** *propoxyphene HCl* 65mg propoxyphene HCl, 32mg caffeine, 389mg aspirin.	ANALGESIC	See *propoxyphene HCl.*
Datril	ANALGESIC	See *acetaminophen.*
daunorubicin HCl **Cerubidine**	ANTINEOPLASTIC **Drug:** Parenterally administered. **Diet:** Encourage ↑ fluids unless otherwise directed. **GI:** N&v, stomach pain. **S/Cond:** Not c̄ lactation. **Other:** Sore throat. **Blood/Serum:** ↑ alk phos, ↑ SGOT, ↑ bilirubin, ↑ uric acid.	
Decadron	CORTICOSTEROID	See listing for *hydrocortisone.*
Deltasone *prednisone*	CORTICOSTEROID	See listing for *hydrocortisone.*
demeclocycline HCl **Declomycin**	TETRACYCLINE **S/Cond:** May be used for SIADH.	See listing for *tetracycline.*

See "Guide to the Use of This Book" p. 5 for explanation of format.

MEDICATION	CLASSIFICATION & DIETARY/RELATED SIGNIFICANCES	
Demerol	ANALGESIC, NARCOTIC	See *meperidine HCl.*
Demulen Contains sucrose[10] *Ethynodiol diacetate- ethinyl estradiol*	CONTRACEPTIVE, oral	See listing for *estrogens.*
Depakene	ANTICONVULSANT	See *valproic acid.*
Depen	HEAVY METAL ANTAGONIST	See *penicillamine.*
Depo-Medrol *methylprednisolone*	CORTICOSTEROID	See listing for *hydrocortisone.*

*deserpidine/
methyclothiazide*
Enduronyl

ANTIHYPERTENSIVE c̄ DIURETIC
Drug: Take c̄ food, 6 hr or more before bedtime. **Diet:** Encourage ↑ fluids unless otherwise directed. **Diet Important:** ↓ Na, ↓ cal, ↑ K diet may be recommended. Avoid natural licorice. **GI:** N&v, diarrhea, cramps. **S/Cond:** Monitor diabetic: ↓ CHO tolerance. **Metab/Phys:** Monitor electrolytes. Blood dyscrasias. **Other:** Dry mouth, ↑ wt, drowsiness, dizziness, anorexia.
Blood/Serum: ↑ uric acid, ↑ Ca, ↓ Na, ↓ K, ↓ Cl, ↓ ℗,

	↓ Mg, ↑ or ↓ glucose, ↓ bicarbonate. **Urinary:** ↑ K, ↑ Cl, ↑ uric acid, ↓ Ca, ↑ Mg, ↑ Na, ↑ bicarbonate.	
desipramine HCl **Norpramin** May contain tartrazine **Pertofrane**	ANTIDEPRESSANT, tricyclic **Drug:** Take c̄ food to ↓ GI upset. **Nutr:** May need ↑ Rib.[13] **GI:** Constipation, epigastric distress. **S/Cond:** Avoid alcohol.[13] Limit caffeine:[19] see Table p. 231. **Metab/Phys:** Blood dyscrasias. Inappropriate ADH syndrome. **Other:** Blurred vision, dry mouth, ↑ wt, dizziness, drowsiness, ↑ appetite for sweets, ↑ or ↓ wt, confusion, altered taste, headache, fatigue. **Blood/Serum:** ↑ or ↓ glucose.	
Desyrel	ANTIDEPRESSANT	See *trazodone HCl.*
dexamethasone **Decadron** **Hexadrol**	CORTICOSTEROID	May contain sulfites. Intensol: 30% alcohol.[7] See *hydrocortisone.*
Dexatrim	APPETITE SUPPRESSANT	See *phenylpropanolamine.*
dexbrompheniramine & pseudoephedrine **Drixoral**	ANTIHISTAMINIC, DECONGESTANT **Drug:** Take c̄ food or H_2O. Swallow cap/tab whole. **S/Cond:** Not c̄ lactation. Avoid alcohol. **Other:** Drowsiness, dry mouth.	

MEDICATION	CLASSIFICATION & DIETARY/RELATED SIGNIFICANCES

dexchlorpheniramine maleate
  Polaramine
  Syrup contains
    sorbitol & 6% alcohol

ANTIHISTAMINIC
  Drug: Take $\bar{c}$ food or H_2O. Swallow tab whole. **GI:** GI distress.
  S/Cond: Not $\bar{c}$ lactation. Avoid alcohol. **Other:** Drowsiness, dizziness, anorexia, dry mouth, confusion, especially in the elderly.

dextroamphetamine sulfate
  Dexedrine
  Elixir: 10% alcohol
    Contains tartrazine

STIMULANT, amphetamine
  Drug: Take 30 min before meals & 6 hr before bedtime. Swallow whole. **GI:** Diarrhea, constipation, GI distress.
  Metab/Phys: Possible hypoglycemia. Monitor growth in children.
  Other: Dry mouth, unpleasant taste, dizziness, anorexia, ↓ wt, tremor, headache.

dextrothyroxine
  Choloxin
  2mg tab contains
    tartrazine[7]

ANTIHYPERLIPEMIC
  Diet Important: ↓ fat, ↓ chol diet may be recommended. Avoid large amounts of goitrogenic foods.[6] See Table p. 236.
  GI: Constipation, dyspepsia, diarrhea. **S/Cond:** Monitor diabetic.
  Metab/Phys: ↑ metabolism. **Other:** Tremors, ↓ wt, altered taste, anorexia, headache.
  Blood/Serum: ↓ chol, ↓ LDL, ↑ T_4, ↑ glucose, ↑ bilirubin, ↑ SGOT, ↑ alk phos.
  Urinary: ↑ glucose.

DiaBeta	ORAL HYPOGLYCEMIC	See *glyburide*.
Diabinese	ORAL HYPOGLYCEMIC	See *chlorpropamide*.
Dialose	STOOL SOFTENER	See *docusate potassium*.
Diamox	DIURETIC, ANTIGLAUCOMA	See *acetazolamide*.

diazepam
  Valium
    ANTIANXIETY, MUSCLE RELAXANT, benzodiazepine
    Drug: Take c̄ food or H_2O. **GI:** N&v, constipation. **S/Cond:** Avoid alcohol. **Other:** Drowsiness, fatigue, dizziness, hiccups, salivary changes, tremors, confusion, ↑ appetite, ↑ wt, blurred vision.

dicloxacillin sodium
  12mg Na/250mg[24]
  Dycill
  Dynapen
  Pathocill
    ANTIBIOTIC, penicillin
    Drug: Take c̄ 8oz H_2O on empty stomach. **Diet:** Acid resistant.[10] **GI:** Nausea, epigastric distress, flatulence, diarrhea. **S/Cond:** Not c̄ lactation.
    Blood/Serum: ↑ SGOT.

MEDICATION	CLASSIFICATION & DIETARY/RELATED SIGNIFICANCES

dicumarol
Dicumarol

ANTICOAGULANT
Diet: Cooking oils c̄ silicone additive ↓ drug absorption. Limit food ↑ in Vit K. Avoid proteolytic enzymes (papain), fried/boiled onions[39] & soybean oil.[8] Supplements: large amounts of Vit A, D, E, K & C alter prothrombin time. **GI:** GI distress, constipation. **S/Cond:** Limit alcohol. Limit caffeine: see Table p. 231. **Other:** Bloating.

dicyclomine HCl
Bentyl

ANTISPASMODIC, ANTISECRETORY
Drug: Take c̄ food or H_2O. **GI:** Constipation, n&v. **S/Cond:** Not c̄ lactation. Limit alcohol. **Other:** Dry mouth, altered taste, bloating, confusion, especially in elderly, dizziness, drowsiness.

Didrex

APPETITE SUPPRESSANT   See **benzphetamine HCl.**

diethylpropion HCl
Tenuate
Tepanil

APPETITE SUPPRESSANT, amphetamine-like
Drug: Take last dose 6 hr before bedtime. Do not crush. **GI:** Constipation. **S/Cond:** Limit caffeine: see Table p. 231. Monitor diabetic: may alter glucose level. **Metab/Phys:** Possible growth suppression in children: ↓ appetite.[4] **Other:** Dry mouth, unpleasant taste.

diethylstilbestrol
Diethylstilbestrol

HORMONE, ESTROGENIC
    Drug: Take c̄ food to ↓ nausea. Take at same time each day. Swallow tab whole. **Nutr:** ↓ absorption of Vit A, D, E, K.[10] **GI:** N&v, abdominal cramps. **S/Cond:** Monitor diabetic: ↓ CHO tolerance. **Metab/Phys:** Edema, jaundice. **Other:** ↑ or ↓ wt, bloating, dizziness, depression.
    Blood/Serum: ↑ alk phos, ↑ bilirubin, ↑ glucose, ↑ T_4, ↑ TG, ↑ phospholipids, ↓ Pyr, ↓ Fol.

diflunisal
Dolobid

ANALGESIC, ANTI-INFLAMMATORY, ANTIPYRETIC
    Drug: Take c̄ food to ↓ GI irritation. Swallow tabs whole.[13] **GI:** GI pain, n&v, diarrhea, constipation, flatulence. **S/Cond:** Caution c̄ lactation. Limit alcohol. **Other:** Headache, fatigue.
    Blood/Serum: ↑ SGOT, ↑ SGPT, ↓ uric acid.
    Urinary: ↑ uric acid, + protein.[3]

MEDICATION	CLASSIFICATION & DIETARY/RELATED SIGNIFICANCES

MEDICATION

digitalis
digitoxin
  Chrystodigin
  Digitoxin
digoxin
  Digoxin
  Lanoxin
  Lime-flavored elixir:
    10% alcohol

CARDIOTONIC, ANTIARRHYTHMIC
    Drug: Take c̄ H_2O ½ hr before or 2 hr after ↑ fiber foods & foods ↑ in Ca.[15] **Diet:** Avoid natural licorice. Maintain diet ↑ in K, ↓ in Na, & adequate in Mg[4] & Ca.[11] Supplements: Ca & Vit D induced hypercalcemia may potentiate drug effects & result in cardiac arrhythmias.[14] **Nutr:** Glucose absorption may be inhibited.
    GI: N&v. **S/Cond:** Caution c̄ herbal teas: see Table p. 232.

dihydroxyaluminum
sodium carbonate
  Rolaids
  53mg Na/tab
  Sodium free Rolaids

ANTACID
    Drug: Take 1–3 hr after meals. **Diet:** Encourage ↑ fluids unless otherwise directed. In hyperphosphatemia, ↓ phosphate diet may be used.[13] **GI:** Constipation c̄ large doses, diarrhea.
    Other: ↓ appetite, ↓ wt, swelling, weakness.

Dilantin

ANTICONVULSANT

See *phenytoin sodium.*

Dilaudid

ANALGESIC

See *hydromorphone HCl.*

Dilor
  dyphylline

BRONCHODILATOR

Elixir: 18% alcohol.
See *dyphylline.*

diltiazem HCl **Cardizem**	ANTIANGINAL, Ca-channel blocker **Drug:** Take drug 1 hr before or 2 hr after meals. **Diet Important:** ↓ cal, ↓ Na. **GI:** Nausea, constipation. **S/Cond:** Avoid alcohol. **Metab/Phys:** Edema, hyperglycemia. **Other:** Dizziness, headache, fatigue, dry mouth, altered taste, anorexia. **Blood/Serum:** ↑ alk phos, ↑ SGOT, ↑ SGPT, ↑ LDH, ↑ CPK.
dimenhydrinate **Dramamine** Liquid: 54% sucrose 5% alcohol	ANTIHISTAMINIC, ANTIEMETIC **Drug:** Take c̄ food or H_2O. Swallow tab whole, unless chewable. **GI:** N&v, epigastric distress, diarrhea. **S/Cond:** Limit alcohol. **Other:** Drowsiness, dry mouth, confusion, especially in elderly, anorexia.
Dimetane **Dimetapp**	ANTIHISTAMINIC See listing for ***brompheniramine maleate.***

diphenhydramine HCl
Benadryl
Elixir: 1.5gm
  sucrose/5ml
  14% alcohol
Spray: 90% alcohol
Caps contain lactose
50mg caps:
  Na bisulfite
	ANTIHISTAMINIC
	Drug: Take c̄ food or H_2O. **GI:** GI distress, constipation. **S/Cond:** Avoid alcohol. **Metab/Phys:** Anemia. **Other:** Sedation, dizziness, disturbed coordination, dry mouth, altered taste.

MEDICATION	CLASSIFICATION & DIETARY/RELATED SIGNIFICANCES

dipyridamole
Persantine

ANTIPLATELET
Drug: Take c̄ 1 cup H_2O, 1 hr before meals. **GI:** GI distress, n&v, diarrhea. **Other:** Dizziness, headache, drowsiness, altered taste.

Disalcid

NSAI   See listing for **salicylsalicylic acid.**

disopyramide
phosphate
Norpace

ANTIARRHYTHMIC
Drug: Take on empty stomach. Swallow cap whole.
GI: Constipation, diarrhea, n&v, GI pain, flatulence. **S/Cond:** Avoid alcohol. **Metab/Phys:** Monitor for hypoglycemia & K imblance.
Other: Dry mouth, blurred vision, anorexia, dizziness.
Blood/Serum: ↑ SGOT, ↑ SGPT, ↑ BUN, ↑ creatinine, ↑ chol, ↑ TG, ↓ K, ↓ glucose, ↓ HCT, ↓ Hb.

disulfiram
Antabuse

ALCOHOL DETERRENT
Drug: Tab may be crushed & mixed c̄ liquid beverages. **Diet:** No alcohol-containing products: sauces, vinegars, cough syrups, or elixirs. **GI:** Dyspepsia. **S/Cond:** Caution c̄ diabetic.[13] **Other:** Garlic or metallic taste, drowsiness, headache, visual problems, fatigue.
Blood/Serum: ↑ chol.[13]

Ditropan

PARASYMPATHOLYTIC   See **oxybutynin Cl.**

Diulo

ANTIHYPERTENSIVE   See **metolazone.**

Diupres	ANTIHYPERTENSIVE c̄ DIURETIC	See *chlorothiazide*. See *reserpine*.
Diuril	ANTIHYPERTENSIVE	See *chlorothiazide*.

docusate calcium
  Surfak

LAXATIVE, STOOL SOFTENER
    Drug: Take c̄ milk/fruit juice. **Diet:** Encourage ↑ fluids unless otherwise directed. Useful c̄ ↓ Na diet. **Nutr:** Alters electrolyte absorption. **GI:** Cramps.
    Blood/Serum: ↑ glucose, ↓ K (long term use).

docusate potassium
  Dialose
  8.7mg K/caps

LAXATIVE, STOOL SOFTENER
    Drug: Take c̄ milk/fruit juice. **Diet:** Encourage ↑ fluids unless otherwise directed. Useful c̄ ↓ Na diet. **Nutr:** Alters electrolyte absorption. **GI:** Cramps.
    Blood/Serum: ↑ glucose, ↓ K (long term use).

docusate sodium
  Colace
  Syrup: 3gm sucrose/5ml[29]
  Sodium: 5mg/100mg tab[2]

LAXATIVE, STOOL SOFTENER
    Drug: Take c̄ H_2O, milk/fruit juice. **Diet:** Encourage fluids unless otherwise directed. **Nutr:** Alters intestinal absorption of H_2O & electrolytes. **GI:** Diarrhea.
    Blood/Serum: ↑ glucose, ↓ K (long term use).

MEDICATION	CLASSIFICATION & DIETARY/RELATED SIGNIFICANCES

Dolene
ANALGESIC — See *propoxyphene HCl.*

Dolobid
ANTI-INFLAMMATORY — See *diflunisal.*

Dolophine
NARCOTIC, ANALGESIC — See *methadone HCl.*

Donnagel
6mg Na/5ml
0.01mg K/5ml
kaolin, pectin,
hyoscyamine sulfate,
atropine sulfate,
scopolamine
hydrobromide opium

ANTIDIARRHEAL
Drug: Oral solution: Mix at room temperature & dilute c̄ milk, chocolate milk or orange juice. **GI:** Constipation. **Other:** Dry mouth, dizziness, altered taste, confusion, especially in elderly. Suspension: 3.8% alcohol.

Donnagel PG
Suspension: 0.72gm sucrose, lactose, glucose & fructose/5ml. 5% alcohol.

Donnatal
phenobarbital,
atropine sulfate,
hyoscyamine sulfate,
scopolamine
hydrobromide

ANTISPASMODIC
Drug: Take ½–1 hr before meals unless otherwise directed.[13] **Nutr:** Elixir: 23% alcohol, & 1.6gm sucrose, glucose, lactose, fructose/5ml. **GI:** N&v, constipation. **S/Cond:** Limit alcohol. **Other:** Dry mouth, altered taste,[10] blurred vision, bloating, drowsiness, dizziness.
Blood/Serum: ↓ bilirubin, ↓ Fol, ↓ B_{12}.[11]

Dopar	ANTIPARKINSONISM	See *levodopa*.
Doriden	HYPNOTIC	See *glutethimide*.

doxepin HCl
Adapin
Sinequan

ANTIDEPRESSANT, tricyclic
    Drug: Take c̄ food to ↓ GI distress. Oral concentrate not compatible c̄ carbonated beverages or high acidic juices. See Table p. 237. **Diet:** ↑ need for Rib. ↑ appetite for sweets. **GI:** Epigastric distress, constipation. **S/Cond:** Limit caffeine:[19] see Table p. 231. Avoid alcohol. **Metab/Phys:** Edema, blood dyacrasias.[3] Inappropriate ADH syndrome. **Other:** Drowsiness, dry mouth, ↑ wt, metallic/sour taste, blurred vision, dizziness.
    Blood/Serum: ↑ or ↓ glucose.

doxorubicin
Adriamycin

ANTINEOPLASTIC
    Drug: Parenterally administered. **Diet:** Encourage ↑ fluids unless otherwise directed. **GI:** N&v, diarrhea, stomach pain. **S/Cond:** Not c̄ lactation. **Other:** Sore throat, mouth sores/ulcers, anorexia, altered taste.
    Blood/Serum: ↑ uric acid.
    Urinary: ↑ uric acid.

MEDICATION	CLASSIFICATION & DIETARY/RELATED SIGNIFICANCES

doxycycline
  Doryx
  Vibramycin
  Contains bisulfite

ANTIBIOTIC, tetracycline
  Drug: Take $\bar{c}$ food, milk[10] or 1 cup fluid. Swallow enteric-coated tab whole. **Diet:** Encourage ↑ fluids unless otherwise directed. **Nutr:** ↓ absorption of Ca, Fe, Mg, Zn, amino acids, & fat; these nutrients may ↓ drug absorption.[11] **GI:** Dysphagia, GI distress, n&v. **Metab/Phys:** ↓ bacterial synthesis of Vit K in intestine. Possible hemolytic anemia. **Other:** Sore mouth, ↑ thirst, anorexia, tiredness.
  Blood/Serum: ↑ BUN.

Dramamine	ANTIEMETIC	See *dimenhydrinate.*
Drixoral	ANTIHISTAMINIC, DECONGESTANT	See *dexbrompheniramine* & *pseudoephedrine.*
Dulcolax	LAXATIVE	See *bisacodyl.*
Duricef	ANTIBIOTIC	See *cefadroxil.*
Dyazide *triamterene $\bar{c}$* *hydrochlorothiazide*	ANTIHYPERTENSIVE, DIURETIC	See *triamterene $\bar{c}$ hydrochlorothiazide.*

Dycill	ANTIBIOTIC	See *dicloxacillin sodium*.
Dymelor	ORAL HYPOGLYCEMIC	See *acetohexamide*.
Dynapen	ANTIBIOTIC	See *dicloxacillin sodium*.

dyphylline — BRONCHODILATOR
Dilor
Elixir: 18% alcohol
Lufyllin
Elixir: 20% alcohol
Lufyllin-400

Drug: Take $\bar{c}$ H$_2$O 1 hr before or 2 hr after meals. Chew chewable tab. Swallow cap/tab whole. **Diet:** Not affected by charbroiled foods.[13] **GI:** N&v, heartburn, epigastric pain, diarrhea. **S/Cond:** Limit caffeine: see Table p. 231. **Metab-/Phys:** Hyperglycemia. **Other:** Headache, agitation.

Dyrenium	DIURETIC	See *triamterene*.
Ecotrin *enteric-coated aspirin*	ANALGESIC	Swallow enteric-coated caps whole. See *acetylsalicylic acid*.

MEDICATION	CLASSIFICATION & DIETARY/RELATED SIGNIFICANCES	
Edecrin	DIURETIC	See *ethacrynic acid.*
Elavil	ANTIDEPRESSANT	See *amitriptyline HCl.*
Elixophyllin	BRONCHODILATOR	See *theophylline.*
Emete-con	ANTINAUSEANT	See *benzquinamide HCl.*
Empirin c̄ codeine	ANALGESIC, NARCOTIC	See *acetylsalicylic acid.* See *codeine.*

enalapril maleate
  Vasotec

ANTIHYPERTENSIVE
  Drug: May take c̄ food. **Diet Important:** Limit salt substitutes & foods ↑ in K. **GI:** Diarrhea, n&v, abdominal pain. **S/Cond:** Limit alcohol. Monitor diabetic: possible hyperglycemia.[2]
  Other: Headache, altered taste.
  Blood/Serum: ↑ BUN, ↑ creatinine, ↑ K, ↓ Na.

encainide HCl
  Enkaid

ANTIARRHYTHMIC
  Diet: Maintain consistent K-balance. **GI:** N&v, constipation, dyspepsia, abdominal pain. **S/Cond:** Caution c̄ diabetic: ↑ glucose level (rare).[10] Limit alcohol. **Other:** Dry mouth, anorexia, altered taste, dizziness, headache.
  Blood/Serum: ↑ alk phos, ↑ SGOT, ↑ SGPT.

Endep	ANTIDEPRESSANT	See *amitriptyline HCl*.
Enduron *methychlothiazide*	DIURETIC	See listing for *hydrochlorothiazide*.
Enduronyl	ANTIHYPERTENSIVE c̄ DIURETIC	See *deserpidine/methyclothiazide*.
Enovid	HORMONE	See listing for **estrogens**.
enteric-coated aspirin	ANALGESIC	See *acetylsalicylic acid*.

Entex LA
guaifenesin & phenylpropanolamine HCl
Entex liquid
guaifenesin, phenylpropanolamine HCl & phenylephrine HCl
5% alcohol

DECONGESTANT, EXPECTORANT
  Drug: Drink H_2O after each dose. Swallow whole. **GI:** GI distress, nausea. **S/Cond.** Not c̄ lactation. Caution c̄ diabetic: prolonged use may cause false + glucose. **Other:** Headache.

Epsom Salts	LAXATIVE, CATHARTIC	See *magnesium sulfate*.

MEDICATION	CLASSIFICATION & DIETARY/RELATED SIGNIFICANCES

Equagesic
*meprobamate,
ethoheptazine &
aspirin*

ANALGESIC
   325mg aspirin.

See *meprobamate.*
See *acetylsalicylic acid.*

Equanil

ANTIANXIETY

See *meprobamate.*

*ergotamine tartrate &
caffeine*
   100mg caffeine/tab
Cafergot

ANTIMIGRAINE
   GI: N&v. **S/Cond:** Avoid alcohol. Monitor diabetic: may impair glucose tolerance. **Metab/Phys:** Edema. **Other:** Drowsiness.

erythromycin
  Bristamycin
  E.E.S.
  E-mycin
  0.75gm sucrose/5ml
  Eryc
  Erythromycin
    suspension
  Ilosone
  Ilotycin
  Pediamycin
  Wyamycin
	ANTIBIOTIC
	    Drug: Swallow enteric-coated tab whole. Chew chewable tab well. Optimal: take on empty stomach 1 hr before or 2 hr after meals. If GI distress, take c̄ meals, not milk. Allow 1 hr before drinking acidic beverages. Less than 5mg Na/dose. Food ↓ absorption.
	    GI: Nausea, epigastric distress, cramps, diarrhea.
	    Metab/Phys: Jaundice.
	    Blood/Serum: ↑ alk phos, ↑ bilirubin, ↑ SGOT, ↑ SGPT.	

Esidrix	ANTIHYPERTENSIVE	See *hydrochlorothiazide.*
Esimil	ANTIHYPERTENSIVE c̄ DIURETIC	See *hydrochlorothiazide.* See *guanethidine monosulfate.*
Eskalith	ANTIMANIC	See *lithium carbonate.*

MEDICATION	CLASSIFICATION & DIETARY/RELATED SIGNIFICANCES

estrogens
(hormone)
Enovid
Evex
Premarin
Provera
(oral contraceptive)
Demulen
Lo/Ovral
Nordette
Norinyl
Ogen
Ovral
Ovulen

HORMONE, ORAL CONTRACEPTIVE

Drug: Take c̄ food at same time each day. ↓ than 5mg Na/dose. **Diet:** Add food ↑ in Fol & Pyr. Supplements: Vit C: 1gm/day will have possible adverse effects: will ↑ serum concentration of estrogen.[9] **Nutr:** ↓ absorption of H_2O soluble vitamins, altered amino acid pattern, altered tryptophan metabolism. **GI:** N&v, colitis. **S/Cond:** Not c̄ lactation. Limit caffeine:[7] see Table p. 231. Monitor diabetic: alters glucose tolerance. **Metab/Phys:** ↓ Ca bone loss,[12] ↑ HDL, ↓ VLDL.[4] Edema, jaundice, pancreatitis. **Other:** ↑ or ↓ wt, bloating, dizziness, weakness.
Blood/Serum: ↑ glucose, ↑ TG, ↑ Vit A, ↑ Vit E, ↓ Vit C, ↑ Fe, ↑ Cu,[1] ↑ phospholipids, ↑ T_4, ↑ alk phos, ↑ bilirubin, ↓ Fol, ↓ Ca, ↓ Mg,[12] ↓ Pyr, ↓ Rib, ↓ Zn.[11]

ethacrynic acid
Edecrin

DIURETIC

Drug: Take c̄ meals, milk, 6 or more hr before bedtime. **Diet:** Need foods ↑ in K & Mg. **GI:** GI distress, n&v, diarrhea. **S/Cond:** Not c̄ lactation. Limit alcohol. Monitor diabetic: ↓ CHO tolerance. **Metab/Phys:** Hypokalemia. **Other:** Anorexia, dizziness. **Blood/Serum:** ↑ glucose, ↑ BUN, ↑ uric acid, ↓ Ca, ↓ Cl, ↓ Mg, ↓ K, ↓ Na.[13]

ethchlorvynol
Placidyl
750mg dose contains tartrazine

HYPNOTIC
Drug: Take c̄ food. **GI:** Nausea. **S/Cond:** Avoid alcohol. **Metab/Phys:** Jaundice. **Other:** Dizziness, drowsiness, blurred vision, aftertaste, weakness.

ethinamate
Valmid

HYPNOTIC
Drug: Take 20 minutes before retiring. **Diet:** No caffeine late in day. See Table p. 231. **GI:** Distress. **S/Cond:** Possible paradoxical excitement (especially in children).[13] Avoid alcohol. **Other:** dizziness, confusion.

ethosuximide
Zarontin

ANTICONVULSANT
Drug: Take c̄ food or milk. **GI:** Diarrhea, n&v, stomach cramps. **Metab/Phys:** Blood dyscrasias. **Other:** Anorexia, ↓ wt, swollen tongue, hiccups, drowsiness.

etidronate disodium
Didronel

CALCIUM REGULATOR
Drug: Take c̄ black coffee, tea, fruit juice, H_2O, on an empty stomach, or at least 2 hr after food. Maintain well-balanced diet c̄ adequate intake of Ca & Vit D.[10] Avoid taking foods ↑ in Ca, or vitamin/mineral supplements c̄ Ca, Fe, Mg, or Al within 2 hr of taking drug.[3] **GI:** Diarrhea, nausea, GI discomfort.
Blood/Serum: ↑ Ⓟ, ↓ alk phos.

See "Guide to the Use of This Book" p. 5 for explanation of format.

MEDICATION	CLASSIFICATION & DIETARY/RELATED SIGNIFICANCES
etoposide **VePesid**	ANTINEOPLASTIC **GI:** N&v, diarrhea, stomatitis. **S/Cond:** Not c̄ lactation. **Metab/Phys:** Blood dyscrasias.[10] **Other:** Anorexia, aftertaste, sore throat. **Blood/Serum:** ↑ bilirubin, ↑ SGOT, ↑ alk phos.
Etrafon *perphenazine & amitriptyline HCl*	ANTIDEPRESSANT, ANTIPSYCHOTIC See listing for *perphenazine.* See listing for *amitriptyline HCl.*
Euthroid *liotrix*	THYROID PREPARATION Orange, brown, grey tabs contain tartrazine. See listing for *thyroid.*
Evex	HORMONE See *estrogens.*
Ex-lax	LAXATIVE See *phenolphthalein.*
famotidine **Pepcid, Pepcid IV**	ANTIULCER **Diet:** Avoid any irritating foods or beverages. **Nutr:** Monitor Vit B_{12} levels. **GI:** Constipation, diarrhea. **S/Cond:** Not c̄ lactation. **Other:** Headache, dizziness.

Fastin	APPETITE SUPPRESSANT	See *phentermine HCl.*
Feldene	NSAI	See *piroxicam.*

fenfluramine HCl
   Pondimin
    APPETITE SUPPRESSANT
    Drug: Take before meals. Swallow cap/tab whole. **GI:** Diarrhea, n&v, abdominal pain, constipation. **S/Cond:** Not $\bar{c}$ lactation. Monitor diabetic: Insulin requirements may be altered.[3]
    Other: Drowsiness, dry mouth, altered taste, tremors, confusion.

fenoprofen
   Nalfon
    ANTIARTHRITIC, NSAI, ANALGESIC
    Drug: Take $\bar{c}$ food. **GI:** Dyspepsia, constipation, n&v, heartburn. **S/Cond:** No alcohol. Not $\bar{c}$ lactation. **Other:** Dry mouth, anorexia, dizziness, confusion.
    Blood/Serum: ↑ SGOT, ↑ LDH, ↑ alk phos, ↑ BUN.[3]

ferrous gluconate
   11.6% elemental Fe
   Fergon
   Fergon Plus
   75mg ascorbic acid & Vit B$_{12}$
ferrous sulfate
   20% elemental Fe
   Feosol
    HEMATINIC
    Drug: Take $\bar{c}$ 8oz of H_2O or juice on an empty stomach. Swallow tabs whole. May take $\bar{c}$ food to prevent irritation; do not take $\bar{c}$ cereals, dietary fiber, tea, coffee, eggs or milk. **Nutr:** Liquid: 3gm sucrose/5ml ($FeSO_4$). Elixir: 0.1mg K/5ml; 3.5mg Na/5ml; 5% alcohol; 44mg Fe/5ml.[31] Vit C ↑ absorption of drug. **GI:** Nausea, constipation, diarrhea. **S/Cond:** Limit alcohol.

106

MEDICATION

Fiberall

Fiorinal
  50mg butalbital,
  325mg aspirin, &
  40mg caffeine

Flagyl

flavoxate HCl
  Urispas

flecainide acetate
  Tambocor

CLASSIFICATION & DIETARY/RELATED SIGNIFICANCES

LAXATIVE   See *psyllium hydrophilic mucilloid.*

ANALGESIC, SEDATIVE
  Drug: Take c̄ food. **GI:** N&v, flatulence, heartburn. **S/Cond:** Limit alcohol. **Other:** Drowsiness, dizziness.
  Blood/Serum: ↑ or ↓ uric acid, dose-related, ↓ T_4, ↑ glucose, ↓ bilirubin.
  Urinary: ↑ glucose (c̄ $CuSO_4$).

ANTIBIOTIC   See *metronidazole.*

ANTISPASMODIC, ANTICHOLINERGIC, urinary
  Drug: Take c̄ H_2O on empty stomach. **GI:** N&v. **Other:** Dry mouth, blurred vision, confusion, especially in elderly.

ANTIARRHYTHMIC
  Diet: Maintain constant K-level in diet. **GI:** N&v, constipation, abdominal pain, diarrhea, flatulence. **S/Cond:** Caution c̄ lactation. **Other:** Dizziness, tremors, altered taste, dry mouth.
  Blood/Serum: ↑ alk phos, ↑ SGOT, ↑ SGPT.

Fleet
  Bisacodyl
  3mg Na/30ml
  enema
  4.4mg Na/118ml
  phosphosoda
  2,217.2mg Na/4 tsp

LAXATIVE
  Diet: Encourage ↑ fluids unless otherwise directed.
  Other: Dehydration.

Flexeril

MUSCLE RELAXANT   See **cyclobenzaprine HCl.**

flucytosine
  Ancobon

ANTIFUNGAL
  GI: N&v, diarrhea. **Metab/Phys:** Anemia. **Other:** Sedation, sore throat.
  Blood/Serum: ↑ SGOT, ↑ SGPT, ↑ alk phos, ↑ LDH, ↑ BUN, ↑ creatinine.

fluorouracil
  Fluorouracil

ANTINEOPLASTIC
  Drug: Parenterally administered. If given orally: Take c̄ H$_2$O, not c̄ acidic beverages. **Diet:** Recommend 100–125gm glucose/day & non-stimulating foods.[15] **Nutr:** ↑ need of Thi. **GI:** N&v, stomatitis, diarrhea, heartburn. **Other** Sore mouth, anorexia, bitter/sour taste, visual changes, weakness.
  Blood/Serum: ↓ albumin, ↑ alk phos, ↑ SGPT, ↑ bilirubin, ↑ LDH.

MEDICATION

CLASSIFICATION & DIETARY/RELATED SIGNIFICANCES

fluoxetine
Prozac

ANTIDEPRESSANT
> **Drug:** Take in the AM s̄ regard to meals. **Diet:** No tryptophan — use ↑ effects.[13] **GI:** Nausea, diarrhea. **Other:** Headache, tremors, dry mouth, anorexia, ↓ wt, drowsiness.

fluphenazine HCl
Prolixin
Elixir: 14% alcohol
  3gm sucrose/5ml
2.5, 5 & 10mg tabs
  contain tartrazine

ANTIPSYCHOTIC
> **Drug:** Take c̄ food or 8oz fluid. Swallow tab whole.
> **Diet:** Supplements: Large doses of ascorbic acid may interfere c̄ drug absorption.[14] **GI:** Constipation. **S/Cond:** Limit alcohol. **Metab/Phys:** Peripheral edema, blood dyscrasias. **Other:** ↑ or ↓ wt, dry mouth, drowsiness, tremors, blurred vision, ↓ appetite. **Urinary:** ↑ bilirubin (false elevation).

flurazepam HCl
Dalmane

SEDATIVE, HYPNOTIC, benzodiazepine
> **Drug:** Swallow cap whole. **GI:** N&v, diarrhea, constipation, heartburn. **S/Cond:** Not c̄ lactation. Limit alcohol. Limit caffeine: see Table p. 231. **Other:** Dry mouth, bitter taste, anorexia, drowsiness, confusion, blurred vision, sore throat & mouth.
> **Blood/Serum:** ↑ SGOT, ↑ SGPT, ↑ alk phos, ↑ bilirubin.

Fortaz   ANTIBIOTIC   See *ceftazidime.*

Fulvicin   ANTIFUNGAL   See *griseofulvin*

Furadantin	ANTIBIOTIC	See ***nitrofurantoin.***

furazolidone
Furoxone
Liquid: sugar free

ANTI-INFECTIVE, ANTIFUNGAL
  Diet: Avoid tyramine-containing foods, especially if on drug more than 5 days. See Table p. 234. **GI:** N&v, colitis. **S/Cond:** Avoid alcohol. **Metab/Phys:** Hypoglycemia. **Other:** Headache.

furosemide
Lasix
Liquid:
  11.5% alcohol

DIURETIC
  Drug: Optimal: Take on an empty stomach. (Food ↓ absorption.[7]) If GI distress, may take $\bar{c}$ food or milk. Do not mix $\bar{c}$ acidic solutions (pH below 5.5). **Diet:** ↓ cal, ↓ Na & fat controlled diet, ↑ in K & Mg, may be recommended.[13] Limit intake of natural licorice. **GI:** Liquid: sorbitol content may ↑ possibility of diarrhea in children. N&v. **S/Cond:** Limit alcohol. Monitor diabetic: ↓ CHO tolerance.[13] **Metab/Phys:** Blood dyscrasias. **Other:** Dizziness, anorexia, dry mouth, peculiar sweet taste.
  Blood/Serum: ↑ glucose, ↑ BUN, ↑ Zn,[11] ↑ uric acid, ↓ Ca, ↓ Mg, ↓ K, ↓ Na, ↓ Cl.
  Urinary: ↑ K, ↑ Na, ↑ Cl, ↑ Mg, ↑ Ca, ↑ glucose.[3]

Gantanol	ANTIBIOTIC	See ***sulfamethoxazole.***
Gantrisin	ANTIBIOTIC	See ***sulfisoxazole.***

See "Guide to the Use of This Book" p. 5 for explanation of format.

MEDICATION	CLASSIFICATION & DIETARY/RELATED SIGNIFICANCES

Garamycin

ANTIBIOTIC   See *gentamicin sulfate.*

Gaviscon
aluminum hydroxide
magnesium trisilicate

ANTACID, ANTIFLATULANT
Drug: Take 1–3 hr after meals c̄ H_2O, milk or juice; chew tab.
Diet: Not c̄ ↓ Na diet. **Nutr:** May ↓ absorption of Vit A & Ⓟ.
GI: Constipation. **Metab/Phys:** Inactivates Thi. **Other:** Dizziness,
anorexia, ↓ wt.
Liquid: 0.3mg sorbitol/5ml, 39mg Na/15ml.
Tab: 1.2gm sucrose & 18mg Na.

Gelusil
magnesium
hydroxide, aluminum
hydroxide &
simethicone
Liquid: 0.7mg Na/5ml
  0.5gm sorbitol/5ml
Tab: 0.8mg Na

ANTACID, ANTIFLATULANT
Drug: Take 1 hr after meals. Chew tab. **Nutr:** May ↓ absorption
of Vit A. Long term use: ↓ P & Ca absorption. **GI:** Constipation.
Metab/Phys: Inactivates Thi.

gemfibrozil **Lopid**	ANTIHYPERLIPEMIC	

Drug: Take ½ hr before meals. **Diet:** Adherence to ↓ fat, cal-controlled diet important. **GI:** <u>Abdominal pain, epigastric distress</u>, diarrhea, n&v, flatulence, constipation. **S/Cond:** Not c̄ lactation. <u>Limit alcohol</u>. Caution c̄ diabetic.[1] **Metab/Phys:** Anemia. **Other:** Headache, dizziness, dry mouth.
Blood/Serum: ↓ K, ↑ SGOT, ↑ alk phos, ↑ SGPT, ↑ LDH, ↑ CPK, ↑ glucose.

gentamicin sulfate **Garamycin** Contains sulfites[7]	ANTIBIOTIC, aminoglycoside	

Drug: Parenterally administered. **Diet:** ↑ fluids unless otherwise directed. **GI:** N&v. **Metab/Phys:** Urinary antibacterial effect ↑ in alkaline urine. **Other:** Anorexia, ↑ thirst, dizziness, ↑ salivation.
Blood/Serum: ↑ BUN, ↑ SGOT, ↑ SGPT, ↑ LDH, ↑ bilirubin, ↑ creatinine, ↓ Mg, ↓ Na, ↓ K, ↓ Ca.
Urinary: ↑ Mg, ↑ K, + for protein.

Geocillin	ANTIBIOTIC	See *carbenicillin indanyl sodium.*
Geopen — IV	ANTIBIOTIC	See *carbenicillin disodium.*

MEDICATION	CLASSIFICATION & DIETARY/RELATED SIGNIFICANCES

glipizide
Glucotrol

ORAL HYPOGLYCEMIC
    Drug: Take 30 minutes before breakfast. **Diet:** Prescribed diet compliance important. **GI:** GI distress, nausea, diarrhea, constipation, heartburn. **S/Cond:** Caution c̄ lactation. Limit alcohol.
    Metab/Phys: Blood dyscrasias. **Other:** Altered taste, dizziness, drowsiness.
    Blood/Serum: ↑ SGOT, ↑ LDH, ↑ alk phos, ↑ BUN, ↑ creatinine, ↓ glucose.

Glucotrol

ORAL HYPOGLYCEMIC   See *glipizide.*

glutethimide
Doridan

HYPNOTIC
    GI: N&v. **S/Cond:** Not c̄ lactation. Avoid alcohol. Limit caffeine.
    Metab/Phys: May ↑ Vit D turnover, alters Ca need.[13] **Other:** Dry mouth, dizziness, blood dyscrasias, drowsiness, blurred vision.

glyburide
DiaBeta
Micronase

ORAL HYPOGLYCEMIC
    Drug: Take before breakfast. **Diet:** Prescribed diet compliance important. **GI:** GI distress, nausea, diarrhea, constipation, heartburn. **S/Cond:** Not c̄ lactation. Limit alcohol. **Metab/Phys:** Blood

dyscrasias. **Other:** Dizziness, drowsiness.
Blood/Serum: ↓ glucose.
Urinary: ↓ glucose.

griseofulvin
Fulvicin
Grifulvin
Grisactin

ANTIFUNGAL
Drug: Take c̄ or after ↑ fatty meal (best absorbed c̄ noon meal); enhances absorption & ↓ GI irritation.[13] **GI:** Nausea, diarrhea, flatulence. **S/Cond:** Avoid alcohol. **Other:** Altered taste, blurred vision, confusion.[1]

guaifenesin
Guaifenesin Syrup
5% alcohol[29]
3.25gm sucrose/5ml

DECONGESTANT, EXPECTORANT
GI: GI distress, nausea. **S/Cond:** Not c̄ lactation. Monitor diabetic.
Other: Headache.

guanethidine sulfate
Ismelin

ANTIHYPERTENSIVE
Drug: Take at same time each day. **Diet Important:** ↓ Na, ↓ cal may be recommended. Avoid natural licorice. **GI:** Diarrhea, nausea. **S/Cond:** Caution c̄ lactation. Limit alcohol.
Metab/Phys: Edema. **Other:** Dizziness, weakness, dry mouth, ↑ wt.
Blood/Serum: ↑ BUN, ↑ creatinine.

MEDICATION	CLASSIFICATION & DIETARY/RELATED SIGNIFICANCES

guanfacine HCl
Tenex

ANTIHYPERTENSIVE, alpha blocker
    Diet Important: Possible Na restriction, wt reduction.
    GI: <u>Constipation</u>, n&v, stomach cramps. **S/Cond:** Avoid alcohol.
    Other: Dizziness, headache, fatigue, drowsiness.

Halcion

SEDATIVE, HYPNOTIC, benzodiazepine   See *triazolam.*

haloperidol
Haldol
  1, 5, 10mg tabs
    contain tartrazine

ANTIPSYCHOTIC
    Drug: Take c̄ food or milk. Do not mix liquid concentrate c̄ coffee
    or tea: drug may precipitate.[13] **GI:** Constipation, diarrhea.
    S/Cond: Avoid alcohol. Not c̄ lactation. **Other:** Dry mouth,
    anorexia, salivation, blurred vision, dizziness.

heparin sodium
Heparin
  7mg Na/2ml vial

ANTICOAGULANT
    Drug: Parenterally administered. No dietary significances.

Hexadrol
  dexamethasone

CORTICOSTEROID   See listing for *hydrocortisone.*

Hiprex

ANTI-INFECTIVE   Contains tartrazine.
                                      See *methenamine hippurate.*

Humulin   ANTIDIABETIC   See *insulin.*

Hydergine
*mixture of
dihydrogenated
ergot alkaloids*

GERIATRIC CEREBRAL STIMULANT
Drug: Dissolve sublingual tablet under tongue. Do not eat, drink, or smoke while tab dissolves.[7] Elixir: 30% alcohol by volume.
GI: Transient nausea, GI distress. **Other:** Possible soreness under tongue.

hydralazine HCl
Apresoline
100mg tabs contain tartrazine

ANTIHYPERTENSIVE, VASODILATOR
Drug: Take c̄ food same time each day.[5] **Diet:** Avoid natural licorice. ↓ cal, ↓ Na, diet may be recommended. Pyr supplementation may correct drug-induced peripheral neuropathy.[12] **GI:** GI distress, constipation. **S/Cond:** Not c̄ lactation. Limit alcohol.
Metab/Phys: Blood dyscrasias. **Other:** Anorexia, dizziness, tremors.
Urinary: ↑ Mn,[13] ↑ Pyr.[11]

MEDICATION

CLASSIFICATION & DIETARY/RELATED SIGNIFICANCES

hydrochlorothiazide
Tablets contain
lactose
Esidrix
HydroDiuril
Oretic

ANTIHYPERTENSIVE, DIURETIC

Drug: Take c̄ food 6 or more hr before bedtime. **Diet Important:** May need ↓ cal, ↓ Na, ↑ K diet. Need foods ↑ in Mg. Avoid natural licorice. Concurrent use c̄ Ca supplements may result in hypercalcemia; c̄ Mg supplement may result in the formation of an insoluble complex. **Nutr:** Long term use: ↑ bone calcium, ↓ absorption Mg. **GI:** N&v, diarrhea, constipation. **S/Cond:** Not c̄ lactation. Limit alcohol. Monitor diabetic: altered insulin requirements.[1] **Metab/Phys:** Monitor electrolytes. Possible hypokalemia. Blood dyscrasias. **Other:** Anorexia, dizziness, dry mouth.
Blood/Serum: ↑ uric acid, ↑ Ca, ↓ Na, ↓ K,[13] ↓ Cl, ↓ Ⓟ, ↓ Mg, ↑ or ↓ glucose,[3] ↑ chol, ↑ LDL, ↑ TG.[13]
Urinary: ↑ Na, ↑ K, ↑ Cl, ↑ bicarbonate, ↓ uric acid,[3] ↑ Pyr, ↑ Thi, ↑ Mg, ↓ Ca, ↑ glucose.[3]

hydrocortisone
Cortef
Cortisol

CORTICOSTEROID

Drug: May take c̄ food. **Diet:** ↑ K, ↓ Na diet may be recommended. Need foods high in Pyr, Vit C, D, Fol, Ca & P.[11]
Nutr: ↓ absorption of Ca & P. **GI:** GI distress. **S/Cond:** Not c̄ lactation. Limit alcohol & caffeine. Monitor diabetic: prolonged use ↓ CHO metabolism. **Metab/Phys:** Monitor electrolytes.[4] Osteoporosis. Possible growth suppression in children.[13] impaired wound

healing.[12] −N balance. Edema. **Other:** Weakness, ↑ wt.
Blood/Serum: ↑ glucose, ↑ TG, ↑ chol, ↑ Na, ↓ K, ↓ Ca, ↓ T$_4$, ↓ uric acid, ↓ Zn.
Urinary: ↑ N, ↑ K, ↑ Ca, ↑ Zn,[11] ↑ Vit C, ↑ uric acid, ↑ glucose.[11]

hydrocortisone sodium succinate **Solu-Cortef**	CORTICOSTEROID	See *hydrocortisone*.
HydroDiuril	ANTIHYPERTENSIVE, DIURETIC	See *hydrochlorothiazide*.
hydromorphone HCl **Dilaudid** 1, 2, 4mg tabs contain tartrazine Syrup: 2.5mg sucrose/5ml	ANALGESIC, NARCOTIC **Drug:** Take 8oz H$_2$O after each dose. **GI:** Constipation, n&v. **S/Cond:** Avoid alcohol. **Metab/Phys:** Delays digestion of food. **Other:** Anorexia, dizziness, drowsiness.	
Hydropres	ANTIHYPERTENSIVE c̄ DIURETIC	See listing for *hydrochlorothiazide*. See listing for *reserpine*.

| MEDICATION | CLASSIFICATION & DIETARY/RELATED SIGNIFICANCES |

MEDICATION

CLASSIFICATION & DIETARY/RELATED SIGNIFICANCES

hydroxyzine
  Atarax
  Vistaril

ANTIANXIETY, ANTINAUSEANT
S/Cond: Avoid alcohol. Not c̄ lactation. **Other:** Drowsiness, dry mouth, tremors, altered taste.

Hygroton

ANTIHYPERTENSIVE, DIURETIC — See *chlorthalidone.*

Hytrin

ANTIHYPERTENSIVE — See *terazosin HCl.*

ibuprofen
  Advil
  Medipren
  Midol 200
  Motrin
  Nuprin
  Rufen

ANTIARTHRITIC, NSAI
Drug: If GI distress, take c̄ food. **GI:** N&v, epigastric distress, bloating, flatulence, constipation, diarrhea. **S/Cond:** Avoid alcohol. Not c̄ lactation. **Metab/Phys:** GI bleeding can cause anemia.[14] Hepatitis, jaundice, blood dyscrasias. **Other:** Loss of appetite, dizziness, visual problems, dry mouth.
Blood/Serum: ↓ glucose, ↑ BUN, ↑ creatinine, ↑ K, ↓ Hb, ↓ HCT, ↑ SGPT, ↑ SGOT.

Ilosone
Ilotycin

ANTIBIOTIC — See *erythromycin.*

imipenem & cilastatin
73.6mg Na/gm [7]
Primaxin

ANTIBIOTIC
Drug: Parenterally administered. **GI:** Diarrhea, n&v, cramps, heartburn. **S/Cond:** Not c̄ lactation. **Other:** ↑ salivation, ↓ wt.
Blood/Serum: ↑ alk phos, ↑ BUN, ↑ K, ↑ Cl, ↓ Na, ↑ SGOT, ↑ SGPT, ↓ Hb, ↓ HCT.
Urinary: + protein.

imipramine HCl
  Tofranil
  Contains sulfites
  Tofranil-PM
  Contains tartrazine

ANTIDEPRESSANT, tricyclic
Drug: If GI distress, take c̄ food. **Diet:** ↑ need for Rib. **GI:** N&v, diarrhea, epigastric distress, stomatitis, cramps, constipation. **S/Cond:** Avoid alcohol. Not c̄ lactation. Limit caffeine:[19] see Table p. 231. **Metab/Phys:** Black tongue, blood dyscrasias, jaundice. Inappropriate ADH syndrome. **Other:** Dry mouth, blurred vision, anorexia, peculiar taste.
Blood/Serum: ↑ or ↓ glucose.

Imodium   ANTIDIARRHEAL   See *loperamide HCl.*

Imuran   IMMUNOSUPPRESSANT   See *azathioprine.*

MEDICATION	CLASSIFICATION & DIETARY/RELATED SIGNIFICANCES

indapamide
Lozol

ANTIHYPERTENSIVE, DIURETIC
   Drug: If GI distress, may take $\bar{c}$ food at same time each day. **Diet Important:** [10] Consider Na, K, cal controlled diet. **GI:** Constipation, GI distress. **S/Cond:** Not $\bar{c}$ lactation. Limit alcohol. Monitor diabetic: may alter glucose tolerance.[13] **Metab/Phys:** Monitor electrolytes. **Other:** Headache, dizziness, muscle cramps, fatigue, agitation, dry mouth, ↓ wt, ↓ appetite.
   Blood/Serum: ↑ BUN, ↑ creatinine, ↑ amylase, ↑ glucose, ↑ uric acid, ↓ Na, ↓ K, ↑ Ca, ↓ Cl, ↓ ℗,[3] ↓ Mg.
   Urinary: ↑ Na, ↑ K, ↓ Ca, ↑ Mg, ↑ Cl, ↑ bicarbonate, ↓ uric acid, ↑ glucose.

Inderal

ANTIHYPERTENSIVE   See **_propranolol HCl._**

Inderide

ANTIHYPERTENSIVE $\bar{c}$ DIURETIC   See listing for **_propranolol HCl._**
    See listing for **_hydrochlorothiazide._**

indomethacin
Indocin

ANTIARTHRITIC, ANTIGOUT, NSAI
   Drug: To ↓ GI distress, take $\bar{c}$ food. **Nutr:** ↓ absorption of amino acids. **GI:** N&v, dyspepsia, diarrhea, constipation, flatulence. **S/Cond:** Not $\bar{c}$ lactation. Limit alcohol. Monitor diabetic: hyperglycemia. **Metab/Phys:** Hyperkalemia. GI bleeding can cause anemia.

		Edema, jaundice, hepatitis. **Other:** Dizziness, headache,[7] ↑ wt, confusion. **Blood/Serum:** ↑ or ↓ glucose, ↑ BUN, ↓ Vit C, ↑ K, ↑ creatinine, ↑ SGOT, ↑ SGPT. **Urinary:** ↑ glucose, + protein, ↓ Na, ↓ K.
Inocor	VASODILATOR	See *amrinone lactate.*
insulin	ANTIDIABETIC	**Diet Important:** Follow appropriate diet. Patient & type of insulin determine meals & cal. **S/Cond:** Limit alcohol. Monitor diabetic for hypo/hyperglycemia. **Blood/Serum:** ↓ glucose, ↓ K, ↓ Mg.[13] **Urinary:** ↓ glucose.[3]
Intal	ANTIASTHMA	20mg lactose/cap. See *cromolyn Na.*
Ionamin	APPETITE SUPPRESSANT	See *phentermine resin.*
Ismelim	ANTIHYPERTENSIVE	See *guanethidine sulfate.*
isocarboxazide Marplan	ANTIDEPRESSANT, MAOI	See listing for *phenelzine sulfate.*

MEDICATION	CLASSIFICATION & DIETARY/RELATED SIGNIFICANCES

isoniazid
INH

ANTITUBERCULAR
Drug: Optimal: Take 1 hr before or 2 hr after meals. May take c̄ food to relieve GI distress. **Diet:** ↑ need of foods ↑ in Fol, Nia, Mg. ↑ need for Pyr: supplement may correct drug-induced peripheral neuritis.[14] May act like MAOI: Avoid foods c̄ histamine & ↑ in pressor amines. See Table p. 234. **Nutr:** May ↓ absorption of Vit B_6, B_{12}, & Ca.[1] **GI:** N&v. **S/Cond:** Caution c̄ lactation. No alcohol.[13] **Metab/Phys:** Possible osteomalacia, anemias.[14]
Other: Possible cracks in lips, dizziness, ↓ appetite.[13]
Blood/Serum: ↑ SGOT, ↑ SGPT, ↑ bilirubin, ↓ Fol.[11]
Urinary: ↑ glucose (false + $CuSO_4$), ↑ Pyr.[1]

Isoptin

ANTIARRHYTHMIC, Ca-channel blocker　　　　See **verapamil HCl.**

Isopto-Carpine

OPHTHALMIC for glaucoma　　　　See **pilocarpine HCl.**

isosorbide dinitrate
Isordil
Sorbitrate

ANTIANGINAL
Drug: Take c̄ 8oz H_2O on empty stomach. Swallow tab/cap whole. Dissolve sublingual tabs under tongue. Chew chewable tabs completely. **GI:** N&v. **S/Cond:** Caution c̄ lactation. Avoid alcohol.[7]
Other: Headache, dizziness, weakness.
Blood/Serum: ↓ chol (can be false reading).[13]

isotretinoin
  Accutane

ANTIACNE
  GI: Abdominal pain. **S/Cond:** Not c̄ lactation. Limit alcohol. Monitor diabetic: alterations in blood sugar concentrations.[13]
  Metab/Phys: Additive toxic effects may result from combination therapy c̄ Vit A or other supplements containing Vit A.[14]
  Other: Dry mouth, fatigue, headache.
  Blood/Serum: ↑ TG, ↑ chol, ↓ HDL, ↑ CPK, ↑ glucose, ↑ uric acid, ↑ LDH.
  Urinary: + protein.

kanamycin sulfate
  Kantrex
  Contains sulfites

ANTIBIOTIC, aminoglycoside
  Diet: Encourage ↑ fluids unless otherwise directed. **GI:** N&v, diarrhea. **Metab/Phys:** Malabsorption of fat, xylose, carotene, Vit A, D, K, & B$_{12}$. **Other:** ↑ thirst, sore mouth, dizziness.
  Blood/Serum: ↑ BUN, ↑ creatinine, ↑ LDH, ↑ SGOT, ↑ SGPT, ↑ bilirubin, ↓ Mg, ↓ K, ↓ Na.
  Urinary: + protein, ↓ specific gravity.

MEDICATION	CLASSIFICATION & DIETARY/RELATED SIGNIFICANCES

ELECTROLYTE

Kaochlor	780mg K/dose (contains tartrazine)
K-Ciel	780mg K/dose, 4% alcohol
K-Lor	585mg K/dose
Klorvess	780mg K/dose, 2.34gm sucrose/5ml
Klotrix	390mg K/dose
K-Lyte/Cl	975mg K/dose, 100mg glucose/tab
K-Tab	390mg K/dose
potassium chloride	See *potassium chloride.*

kaolin & pectin	ANTIDIARRHEAL
Kaopectate	**Metab/Phys:** Replace fluid loss, monitor electrolytes.

Keflex	ANTIBIOTIC, cephalosporin	Suspension: 3gm sucrose/5ml.
		See *cephalexin monohydrate.*

Keflin	ANTIBIOTIC	99mg Na/gm.
		See *cephalothin sodium.*

Kefzol	ANTIBIOTIC	48.3mg Na/gm.
		See *cefazolin sodium.*

Kenalog-40	CORTICOSTEROID	See ***triamcinolone.***

ketoconazole
Nizoral
ANTIFUNGAL
Drug: Take c̄ food to ↓ n&v. **GI:** N&v, abdominal pain, diarrhea.
S/Cond: Avoid alcohol. Not c̄ lactation. **Metab/Phys:** Anemia.
Other: Headache, dizziness.
Blood/Serum: ↑ SGPT, ↑ SGOT, ↑ alk phos, ↑ bilirubin.

ketoprofen
Orudis
ANTIARTHRITIC, NSAI
Drug: Optimal: Take 30 min before meals or 2 hr after. Take c̄ 8oz H_2O. **GI:** Dyspepsia, nausea, diarrhea, constipation, flatulence.
S/Cond: Avoid alcohol. Not c̄ lactation. **Other:** Anorexia, headache, dizziness, drowsiness, dry mouth, fluid retention, ↑ wt.
Blood/Serum: ↑ LDH, ↑ BUN, ↓ Na, ↑ SGOT, ↑ SGPT, ↓ Hb, ↓ HCT, ↑ alk phos.

Klonopin	ANTICONVULSANT	See ***clonazepam.***

See "Guide to the Use of This Book" p. 5 for explanation of format.

MEDICATION	CLASSIFICATION & DIETARY/RELATED SIGNIFICANCES

K-Phos Neutral
diabasic sodium phosphate & potassiun phosphate
Tab contains 250mg P, 45mg K, 298mg Na

ACIDIFIER, PHOSPHOROUS PREPARATION
Drug: Take c̄ 8oz H_2O after meals or c̄ food to lessen stomach upset or laxative action. Drink 8oz of H_2O each waking hr unless otherwise directed. Take exactly as directed. **Diet:** K or Na controlled diet may be indicated. **GI:** Diarrhea, n&v, stomach pain. **Metab/Phys:** Monitor electrolytes. **Other:** Dizziness, ↑ thirst, ↑ wt (pedal edema), fatigue.[13]
Blood/Serum: ↓ Ca, ↑ P.[7]
Urinary: ↓ Ca.[1]

K-Phos Original

Sodium-free. 500mg tab: 114mg P; 144mg K/tab.

labetalol HCl
Normodyne
Trandate

ANTIHYPERTENSIVE, beta blocker
Drug: Take c̄ food. **Diet:** ↓ Na, ↓ cal diet may be prescribed. **GI:** N&v, dyspepsia. **S/Cond:** Caution c̄ lactation. Limit alcohol. Monitor diabetic: may mask symptoms of hypoglycemia. **Other:** Dizziness, altered taste, headache.
Blood/Serum: ↑ BUN, ↑ SGOT, ↑ SGPT, ↓ HDL, ↑ TG, ↑ K,[1] ↑ uric acid, ↓ glucose.

lactulose
Cephulac
Chronulac
Contains
  2.2gm galactose,
  1.2gm lactose
  & 1.2gm other
  sugars/15ml
	ANTIHYPERAMMONEMIC, LAXATIVE
	Drug: May be mixed c̄ fruit juice, milk, H_2O, or citrus-flavored carbonated beverage. **Diet:** Encourage ↑ fluids unless otherwise directed. **Diet Important:** Not c̄ ↓ galactose diet. **GI:** Constipation, cramps, flatulence, nausea, diarrhea, belching. **S/Cond:** Monitor diabetic. For elderly patients on long-term therapy: monitor electrolytes. **Metab/Phys:** ↓ blood ammonia & ↑ patient tolerance to protein.[10]	

Lanoxin	CARDIOTONIC	See ***digoxin***.
Larodopa	ANTIPARKINSONISM	See ***levodopa***.
Larotid	ANTIBIOTIC	See ***amoxicillin***.
Lasix	DIURETIC	See ***furosemide***.
Ledercillin-VK	ANTIBIOTIC	See ***penicillin V potassium***.
Lente Insulin	ANTIDIABETIC	See ***insulin***.
Leukeran	ANTINEOPLASTIC	See ***chlorambucil***.

See "Guide to the Use of This Book" p. 5 for explanation of format.

MEDICATION	CLASSIFICATION & DIETARY/RELATED SIGNIFICANCES
levodopa **Dopar** Contains tartrazine **Larodopa**	ANTIPARKINSONISM **Drug:** Food can be taken 15 minutes after drug. Not c̄ ↑ protein foods; i.e. milk, cheese, meat, etc. **Diet:** Limit Pyr to 10 mg/day:[14] a supplement dose as low as 5mg may abolish drug's effect. ↑ need of Vit C & B$_{12}$. **Nutr:** Need 0.5gm high biological value protein/Kg body wt/day. **GI:** Epigastric distress, n&v. **S/Cond:** Not c̄ lactation. Avoid caffeine: see Table p. 231. Monitor diabetic: may alter blood glucose.[13] **Other:** Anorexia, dry mouth, altered taste,[37] dizziness, tremors, anxiety. **Blood/Serum:** ↑ BUN, ↑ SGOT, ↑ SGPT, ↑ alk phos, ↑ bilirubin, ↑ LDH, ↓ Hb, ↓ HCT.[3] **Urinary:** ↑ Na, ↑ K, ↑ glucose, ↑ uric acid, ↑ glucose (false + CuSo$_4$).
levodopa & carbidopa **Sinemet**	ANTIPARKINSONISM **Drug:** May take c̄ food to lessen n&v. **Diet:** No need to limit high Pyr foods. **GI:** N&v, flatulence. **S/Cond:** Not c̄ lactation. Monitor diabetic: may alter blood glucose. **Metab/Phys:** Edema. **Other:** Dry mouth, ↑ or ↓ wt, bitter taste, blurred vision. **Blood/Serum:** ↑ BUN, ↑ SGOT, ↑ SGPT, ↑ LDH, ↑ alk phos, ↑ bilirubin. **Urinary:** ↑ uric acid, ↑ or ↓ glucose.

levorphanol tartrate **Levo-Dromoran**	ANALGESIC, NARCOTIC	Oral solution: 2mg sucrose/5ml. See *morphine.*
levothyroxine sodium	THYROID PREPARATION	See listing for *thyroid.*

Librax
*chlordiazepoxide HCl
& clindinium bromide*
 ANTISPASMODIC, ANTISECRETORY, ANTICHOLINERGIC, benzodiazepine
 Drug: Take on empty stomach. **GI:** Constipation, bloating, nausea. **S/Cond:** Not c̄ lactation. Avoid alcohol. **Metab/Phys:** Blood dyscrasias. **Other:** Dry mouth, drowsiness, confusion, blurred vision, dizziness.

Libritabs **Librium**	ANTIANXIETY, benzodiazepine	See *chlordiazepoxide.*

Limbitrol ANTIANXIETY, benzodiazepine, ANTIDEPRESSANT, tricyclic
 See listing for *chlordiazepoxide.* See listing for *amitriptyline.*

*lincomycin HCl
 monohydrate*
Lincocin
 ANTIBIOTIC
 Drug: Take c̄ 8oz H_2O 1 hr before or 2 hr after meal.[13]
 GI: <u>Diarrhea</u>, n&v, flatulence,[13] bloating. **Other:** Altered taste, ↓ wt, ↑ thirst.

Lioresal	ANTISPASMODIC	See *baclofen.*

See "Guide to the Use of This Book" p. 5 for explanation of format.

130

MEDICATION	CLASSIFICATION & DIETARY/RELATED SIGNIFICANCES

liothyronine sodium
  Cytomel

THYROID HORMONE
   Drug: Dosage in range of daily hormonal requirements are ineffective for wt loss.[10] **Diet:** Avoid large amounts of goitrogenic foods: see Table p. 236. **GI:** Diarrhea, vomiting. **S/Cond:** Caution c̄ lactation. Monitor diabetic: hyperglycemia. **Other:** Altered taste, ↓ wt, headache.
   Blood/Serum: ↑ glucose, ↓ T_4.
   Urinary: + glucose.[3]

liotrix
  Euthroid
  Thyrolar

THYROID PREPARATION   See listing for **thyroid.**

lisinopril
  Prinivil
  Zestril

ANTIHYPERTENSIVE
   GI: Diarrhea, vomiting. **Other:** Dizziness, headache.
   Blood/Serum: ↑ BUN, ↑ K.[9]

lithium carbonate
   Eskalith
   Lithane contains
   tartrazine
   Lithobid
   Lithonate
   Lithotabs

ANTIMANIC
   Drug: Take c̄ food. Drink 2–3qts H_2O, fluids/day. Swallow tab whole. **Diet:** Avoid dietary extremes. <u>Important: constancy of daily Na intake is key to stable lithium levels.</u> Be aware of the Na content of common foods. **GI:** N&v, diarrhea. **S/Cond:** Not c̄ lactation. Limit caffeine: see Table p. 231. **Metab/Phys:** ↓ Ca uptake by bone.[11] Alters glucose tolerance. Monitor electrolytes. Edema.[9] **Other:** Metallic taste, ↑ wt, ↑ thirst, dry mouth, blurred vision,[1] drowsiness, dizziness, altered taste/smell,[37] aftertaste.
   Blood/Serum: ↑ Mg, ↓ T_4.
   Urinary: ↑ glucose, albumin.[3]

Lithostat

ANTI-INFECTIVE, urinary   See **acetohydroxamic acid.**

Lomotil
   diphenoxylate HCl
   c̄ atropine sulfate
   Liquid: 1.755gm
      sorbitol/5ml

ANTIDIARRHEAL
   Drug: May take c̄ food.[13] **GI:** N&v, bloating. **S/Cond:** Avoid alcohol. Caution c̄ lactation. **Metab/Phys:** Monitor fluids & electrolytes, especially in children. **Other:** Anorexia, dry mouth, sore/swollen gums, dizziness, drowsiness.
   Blood/Serum: ↑ amylase.

MEDICATION	CLASSIFICATION & DIETARY/RELATED SIGNIFICANCES

lomustine
  Cee Nu

ANTINEOPLASTIC
  Drug: Take on empty stomach to ↓ nausea. **GI:** N&v, stomatitis.
  S/Cond: Not c̄ lactation. **Metab/Phys:** Anemias. **Other:** ↓ appetite.
  Blood/Serum: ↑ alk phos, ↑ SGOT, ↑ SGPT, ↑ bilirubin.

Loniten   ANTIHYPERTENSIVE   See *minoxidil.*

Lo/Ovral   CONTRACEPTIVE, oral   See listing for *estrogen.*
  ethynodiol diacetate
  c̄ mestranol

loperamide HCl
  Imodium
  5.25% alcohol/5ml

ANTIDIARRHEAL
  GI: Abdominal pains, constipation, bloating, n&v.[7] **S/Cond:** Caution
  c̄ lactation. **Other:** Dry mouth, drowsiness, dizziness.

Lopid   ANTIHYPERLIPEMIC   See *gemfibrozil.*

Lopressor   ANTIHYPERTENSIVE   See *metoprolol tartrate.*

lorazepam
  Ativan

ANTIANXIETY, benzodiazepine
  Drug: Swallow tabs whole. **S/Cond:** Avoid alcohol. Limit caffeine:
  see Table p. 231. **Other:** Sedation, dizziness, weakness, altered
  appetite, ↑ wt,[4] blurred vision, headache, tiredness.
  Blood/Serum: ↑ LDH

Lorelco	ANTIHYPERLIPEMIC	See *probucol.*
lovastatin **Mevacor**	ANTIHYPERLIPEMIC	

    Drug: Dose: if single take c̄ evening meal; if twice daily c̄ meals.[41]
    Diet Important: ↓ fat, ↓ chol, ↓ cal diet may be prescribed.
    GI: Constipation, flatulence, abdominal pain, diarrhea, dyspepsia, heartburn, nausea. **S/Cond:** Not c̄ lactation. **Other:** Headache, blurred vision, weakness.
    Blood/Serum: ↑ CPK, ↓ TG, ↓ LDL, ↑ HDL.

loxapine HCl **Loxitane**	ANTIPSYCHOTIC	

    Drug: Take c̄ food or H_2O. **GI:** Constipation, n&v. **S/Cond:** Avoid alcohol. Not c̄ lactation. **Metab/Phys:** Edema. **Other:** Drowsiness, dizziness, confusion, ↑ or ↓ wt, blurred vision.
    Blood/Serum: ↑ SGOT, ↑ SGPT.

Lozol	ANTIHYPERTENSIVE	See *indapamide.*
Ludiomil	ANTIDEPRESSANT	See *maprotiline HCl.*

Lufyllin
Lufyllin-400
  dyphylline
	BRONCHODILATOR
	    Elixir — 20% alcohol.
		See *dyphylline.*

MEDICATION	CLASSIFICATION & DIETARY/RELATED SIGNIFICANCES

Maalox
aluminum hydroxide & magnesium hydroxide
Suspension: 1.4mg Na
Tab: 0.7mg Na

ANTACID
Drug: Take $\bar{c}$ H_2O. Liquid: take between meals & at bedtime. Tab: Chew well. **Nutr:** May ↓ absorption of Vit A. Long term use: ↓ absorption of Ⓟ & Ca.

Maalox Plus
aluminum & magnesium hydroxide plus simethicone

ANTACID, ANTIFLATULENT

See *Maalox.*
Suspension: 0.225gm sorbitol/5ml.
0.8mg Na/tab.
27mg Na/100ml.

Macrodantin
nitrofurantoin macrocrystals

ANTIBIOTIC, urinary

Capsules contain lactose.
See *nitrofurantoin.*

magnesium sulfate
Epsom Salts

LAXATIVE, CATHARTIC
Drug: Mix in H_2O & take on empty stomach. **Diet:** Encourage ↑ fluids unless otherwise directed. **GI:** N&v, cramping, diarrhea. **Other:** Bitter taste, ↑ thirst, dizziness.

Mandelamine

ANTIBIOTIC, urinary

See *methenamine mandelate.*

Mandol	ANTIBIOTIC	See ***cefamandole nafate.***

mannitol
Osmitrol

DIURETIC, DIAGNOSTIC
GI: N&v. **Metab/Phys:** Possible fluid and electrolyte imbalance.
Other: Thirst, lethargy, headache.

maprotiline HCl
Ludiomil
Contains lactose

ANTIDEPRESSANT
Drug: Take c̄ food to ↓ GI distress. **Nutr:** ↑ need for Rib.[3]
GI: Constipation, nausea, diarrhea, heartburn. **S/Cond:** Avoid alcohol. Limit caffeine: see Table p. 231. **Metab/Phys:** Edema.
Other: Dry mouth, blurred vision, drowsiness, tremors, bitter taste, ↑ or ↓ wt,[3] ↑ salivation, fatigue.
Blood/Serum: ↑ or ↓ glucose.[3]

Marax
theophylline,
ephedrine sulfate &
hydroxyzine HCl
Syrup: 5% alcohol

BRONCHODILATOR
Drug: Take c̄ 8oz of H_2O on empty stomach. Swallow tab whole.
GI: Gastric irritation. **Metab/Phys:** Avoid alcohol. Limit xanthine-containing beverages: see Table p. 231. **Other:** Drowsiness, dizziness, weakness, dry mouth, headache.[3]
Blood/Serum: ↑ uric acid, ↑ glucose, ↑ bilirubin.
Urinary: albumin.

Marplan ***isocarboxazide***	ANTIDEPRESSANT, MAOI	See listing for ***phenelzine sulfate.***

MEDICATION	CLASSIFICATION & DIETARY/RELATED SIGNIFICANCES

Matulane   ANTINEOPLASTIC   See *procarbazine HCl.*

Maxzide   ANTIHYPERTENSIVE, DIURETIC   See *triamterene* & *hydrochlorothiazide.*

mazindol
Sanorex

ANTINEOPLASTIC — APPETITE SUPPRESSANT
> **Drug:** Take on empty stomach. Do not crush or chew.
> **GI:** Constipation, n&v. **S/Cond:** Avoid alcohol. Monitor diabetic: Insulin requirements may be altered.[3] **S/Cond:** Dizziness, drowsiness, unpleasant taste, dry mouth, blurred vision, weakness.

Mebaral   ANTICONVULSANT   See *mephobarbital.*

meclizine HCl
Antivert
Bonine

ANTINAUSEANT, ANTIVERTIGO
> **Drug:** Take c̄ food or milk, **S/Cond:** Limit alcohol.
> **Other:** Drowsiness, dry mouth, blurred vision.

meclofenamate sodium
Meclomen

NSAI, ANTIARTHRITIC
> **Drug:** Take c̄ food. **GI:** Diarrhea, n&v, abdominal pain, flatulence, heartburn. **S/Cond:** Avoid alcohol.[13] Not c̄ lactation.
> **Metab/Phys:** Fecal blood loss of 1–2ml/day per 300mg dose. Edema. **Other:** Blurred vision, anorexia, drowsiness, headache.
> **Blood/Serum:** ↑ SGOT, ↑ SGPT, ↑ BUN, ↑ alk phos, ↑ creatinine,[3] ↓ HCT, ↓ Hb.

Medipren	ANTIARTHRITIC	See *ibuprofen.*
Medrol *methylprednisolone*	CORTICOSTEROID	See listing for *hydrocortisone.*

medroxyprogesterone acetate
  Provera
  HORMONE
  Drug: Take at same time each day. **S/Cond:** Monitor diabetic: ↓ glucose tolerance. **Metab/Phys:** Edema. **Other:** ↑ or ↓ wt, altered appetite, weakness, visual problems.
  Blood/Serum: ↑ alk phos, ↑ SGOT, ↑ SGPT, ↑ bilirubin.

mefenamic acid
  Ponstel
  ANALGESIC, NSAI
  Drug: Take c̄ food. **GI:** GI ulceration, n&v, diarrhea, constipation, flatulence, bloating. **S/Cond:** Not c̄ lactation. Avoid alcohol. Monitor diabetic: ↑ insulin requirement. **Metab/Phys:** Anemia.
  Other: Anorexia, blurred vision, drowsiness, dizziness, headache.

Mefoxin	ANTIBIOTIC	See *cefoxitin.*

megestrol acetate
  Megace
  Progestin
  ANTINEOPLASTIC, HORMONE
  GI: Abdominal pain, nausea. **S/Cond:** Not c̄ lactation. Monitor diabetic: ↓ glucose tolerance. **Other:** Altered appetite, ↑ or ↓ wt, weakness, headache.
  Blood/Serum: ↑ alk phos.

See "Guide to the Use of This Book" p. 5 for explanation of format.

MEDICATION	CLASSIFICATION & DIETARY/RELATED SIGNIFICANCES

Mellaril

ANTIPSYCHOTIC   See *thioridazine HCl.*

melphalan
Alkeran

ANTINEOPLASTIC
Drug: Encourage ↑ fluids unless otherwise directed. **GI:** Black, tarry stools, n&v. **S/Cond:** Not c̄ lactation. **Metab/Phys:** Anemia, edema. **Other:** ↓ appetite, mouth sores/ulcers.
Blood/Serum: ↑ uric acid.
Urinary: ↑ uric acid.

meperidine HCl
Demerol

ANALGESIC, NARCOTIC
Drug: Parenterally or orally administered. Dilute syrup in 4oz H_2O. Take c̄ H_2O. May contain sulfites. **GI:** N&v, constipation, stomach cramps. **S/Cond:** Avoid alcohol. **Other:** Drowsiness, dizziness, sedation, dry mouth, ↓ appetite, weakness.
Urinary: ↑ amylase, ↑ lipase.

mephenytoin
Mesantoin
Tab contains lactose[10]

ANTICONVULSANT
Drug: Take c̄ food or milk.[13] **Diet:** Pyr & Fol supplements may ↓ drug's effects.[14] **GI:** Nausea, constipation, diarrhea.
S/Cond: Caution c̄ lactation. Avoid alcohol. Monitor diabetic.
Metab/Phys: Edema, blood dysrasias. **Other:** Drowsiness, dizziness, tremors, headache.
Blood/Serum: ↑ glucose, ↑ alk phos.[3]

mephobarbital **Mebaral**	SEDATIVE, HYPNOTIC, ANTICONVULSANT	See listing for ***phenobarbital.***

meprobamate
Equanil Wyseals
400mg tab: tartrazine
Miltown

ANTIANXIETY
GI: N&v, diarrhea. **S/Cond:** Caution c̄ lactation. Avoid alcohol. **Metab/Phys:** Blood dyscrasias.[7] **Other:** Drowsiness, dizziness, anorexia, slurred speech, weakness.

mercaptopurine
Purinethol

ANTINEOPLASTIC
Diet: Encourage ↑ fluids unless otherwise directed. **GI:** Stomatitis, n&v, diarrhea, stomach pain. **S/Cond:** Avoid alcohol. Not c̄ lactation. **Other:** Fatigue, anorexia, headache.
Blood/Serum: ↑ BUN, ↑ SGOT, ↑ SGPT, ↑ HCT, ↑ bilirubin, ↑ creatinine, ↑ LDH, ↑ uric acid.
Urinary: ↑ uric acid.

mesoridazine
Serentil
Concentrate:
0.6% alcohol

ANTIPSYCHOTIC
Drug: Take c̄ food, milk or H_2O. Swallow tab whole. Liquid: dilute each dose in fruit juice or other acidic beverages (i.e. carbonated beverages). **Nutr:** ↑ need for Rib.[11] **GI:** Constipation, n&v.
S/Cond: Avoid alcohol. **Other:** Dry mouth, dizziness, drowsiness, weakness, tremors, blurred vision.
Urinary: ↑ bilirubin (false elevation).

See "Guide to the Use of This Book" p. 5 for explanation of format.

140

MEDICATION	CLASSIFICATION & DIETARY/RELATED SIGNIFICANCES

Metamucil　　　　　LAXATIVE　　　　See *psyllium.*

metaproterenol sulfate　　BRONCHODILATOR
Alupent　　　　　　**GI:** N&v. **S/Cond:** Caution c̄ diabetics. Caution c̄ lactation.
Metaprel　　　　　　**Other:** Tremors, bad taste.
Liquid contains
sulfites

methadone HCl　　ANALGESIC, NARCOTIC
Methadone　　　　**Drug:** Take c̄ juice or H_2O. **GI:** Constipation, n&v. **S/Cond:** Avoid
Oral solution　　　alcohol. **Other:** Drowsiness, dry mouth, dizziness, anorexia.
contains sorbitol,
8% alcohol
Dolophine

methenamine hippurate　ANTIBIOTIC, urinary, ANTISPASMODIC
Hiprex　　　　　　**Drug:** Take after meals c̄ 4oz H_2O. Maintain acidic urine of pH 5.5
Contains tartrazine　or below;[13] see Table p. 238. Dissolve granule form in 4oz H_2O,
Urex　　　　　　stir well; swallow enteric-coated tabs whole. **Diet:** Encourage fluids
　　　　　　　　　unless otherwise directed. **GI:** Nausea, GI distress.[13]
　　　　　　　　　Blood/Serum: ↑ SGOT, ↑ SGPT.[3]

methenamine mandelate **Mandelamine**	ANTIBIOTIC, urinary No altered lab values.	See listing for ***methenamine hippurate***.
methicillin sodium **Staphcillin** 67–71mg Na/gm	ANTIBIOTIC, penicillin **Drug:** Parenterally administered. **GI:** Diarrhea, vomiting, flatulence, stomatitis. **S/Cond:** Caution c̄ lactation.[13] **Metab/Phys:** Blood dyscrasias. **Other:** Anorexia, glossitis. **Urinary:** albumin.	
methimazole **Tapazole**	ANTITHYROID **Drug:** Take consistently in relation to meals every day. **GI:** N&v, epigastric distress. **S/Cond:** Not c̄ lactation. **Other:** altered taste. **Blood/Serum:** ↑ LDH, ↑ SGPT, ↑ SGOT, ↑ alk phos, ↑ bilirubin.[13]	
methocarbamol **Robaxin**	MUSCLE RELAXANT **Drug:** Oral administration: Tablets may be crushed, mixed c̄ food, liquid. **GI:** GI upset: injectable form only. Nausea. **S/Cond:** Avoid alcohol. Not c̄ lactation. **Other:** Drowsiness, anorexia, metallic taste.	

MEDICATION	CLASSIFICATION & DIETARY/RELATED SIGNIFICANCES

methotrexate
Methotrexate

ANTINEOPLASTIC, ANTIPSORIATRIC
Diet: Encourage ↑ fluids unless otherwise directed. Supplements: PABA may ↑ toxicity; Fol may ↓ drug response.[14] **Nutr:** May ↓ absorption of fat, Vit B_{12}, lactose, Fol, carotene, chol.[13] Milky meals may ↓ drug absorption. **GI:** Stomatitis, n&v, distention, diarrhea, steatorrhea, GI ulceration. **S/Cond:** Avoid alcohol. **Metab/Phys:** Blood dyscrasias. **Other:** Anorexia, mouth sores/ulcers. **Blood/Serum:** ↑ uric acid, ↑ SGOT.[13] **Urinary:** ↑ uric acid.

methyclothiazide
Aquatensen
Enduron

ANTIHYPERTENSIVE, DIURETIC   See listing for **hydrochlorothiazide.**

methyldopa
Aldomet
IV contains sulfites

ANTIHYPERTENSIVE
Diet Important: ↓ Na, ↓ cal diet may be recommended. ↑ need of Vit B_{12} & Fol. Avoid natural licorice. **GI:** Diarrhea, nausea. **S/Cond:** Limit alcohol. **Metab/Phys:** Edema, possible hemolytic anemia. **Other:** Dry mouth, drowsiness, ↑ wt, depression. **Blood/Serum:** ↑ alk phos,[3] ↑ SGOT, ↑ SGPT, ↑ bilirubin, ↑ uric acid, ↑ BUN, ↑ K, ↑ Na.[13]

methylphenidate HCl **Ritalin**	PSYCHOSTIMULANT	

Drug: Take ½ hour before meals and no later than 6 PM. Swallow tab whole. **GI:** Nausea, stomach pain. **S/Cond:** Caution c̄ lactation. **Metab/Phys:** ↓ growth rate, ↓ wt in hyperactive children: diminishes c̄ time. **Other:** Dizziness, drowsiness, ↓ wt, anorexia, headache.

methylprednisolone **Depo-Medrol** **Medrol**	CORTICOSTEROID	See listing for *hydrocortisone.*

methysergide maleate **Sansert** Contains tartrazine, lactose, sucrose	ANTIMIGRAINE

Drug: Take c̄ food or milk. **Diet:** ↓ Na diet may be recommended. Monitor cal intake. **GI:** Indigestion, n&v, diarrhea, heartburn,[7] abdominal pain, constipation. **S/Cond:** Not c̄ lactation. Avoid alcohol. **Metab/Phys:** Edema. **Other:** Anorexia, ↑ or ↓ wt, dizziness, drowsiness.
Blood/Serum: ↑ BUN.

metoclopramide HCl **Reglan**	GI STIMULANT

Drug: Take ½ hour before meals & at bedtime.[9] **GI:** Nausea, diarrhea. **S/Cond:** Caution c̄ lactation. Avoid alcohol. Monitor diabetics: may alter insulin requirements.[3] **Other:** Drowsiness, dizziness, headache, sedation, fatigue, fluid retention.

MEDICATION	CLASSIFICATION & DIETARY/RELATED SIGNIFICANCES

metolazone
Diulo
Zaroxolyn

DIURETIC
Drug: Take in AM after breakfast or last dose before 6 PM.
Diet: High K diet may be recommended. **GI:** Constipation, nausea, bloating. **S/Cond:** Not c̄ lactation. Limit alcohol. Monitor diabetic.
Metab/Phys: Monitor electrolytes (possible hypokalemia, hyponatremia). Hypochloremic alkalosis, blood dyscrasias. **Other:** Dry mouth, anorexia, dizziness, drowsiness.
Blood/Serum: ↑ or ↓ glucose, ↑ uric acid, ↑ Ca, ↓ Na, ↓ K, ↓ Cl, ↓ bicarbonate, ↑ BUN, ↑ creatinine, ↓ or ↑ Mg, ↓ Ⓟ.
Urinary: ↑ glucose, ↑ K, ↑ Na, ↑ Cl, ↑ bicarbonate, ↑ uric acid, ↑ Mg, ↓ Ca,[13] ↑ Ⓟ.

metoprolol tartrate
Lopressor

ANTIHYPERTENSIVE, beta blocker
Drug: Take c̄ food: enhances absorption. **Diet Important:** ↓ Na, ↓ cal may be recommended. **GI:** Diarrhea, GI pain, flatulence, constipation, heartburn. **S/Cond:** Not c̄ lactation. Caution c̄ diabetic: may mask symptoms of hypoglycemia.[13] **Other:** Mental confusion, fatigue, dizziness, dry mouth.
Blood/Serum: ↑ BUN, ↑ SGOT, ↑ SGPT, ↑ alk phos, ↓ HDL,[1] ↑ TG, ↑ K, ↑ uric acid.[1]

metronidazole **Flagyl**	ANTIBIOTIC, AMEBACIDAL, ANTITRICHOMONAL **Drug:** Take c̄ food. **GI:** N&v, diarrhea, epigastric distress, constipation, stomatitis. **S/Cond:** Not c̄ lactation. Avoid alcohol. **Metab/Phys:** Disulfiram-like reaction. **Other:** Anorexia, dizziness, drowsiness, metallic taste, dry mouth, headache. **Blood/Serum:** ↓ SGOT.
Mevacor	ANTIHYPERLIPEMIC See *lovastatin*.
mexiletine HCl **Mexitil**	ANTIARRHYTHMIC **Drug:** Take c̄ food, milk or immediately after meals.[13] **Diet:** Avoid diet changes which drastically acidify or alkalinize urine: see Table p. 238. **GI:** Nausea, lactation. **Other:** Appetite changes, dizziness, tremors, weakness. **Blood/Serum:** ↑ SGOT.
mezlocillin **Mezlin** 43mg Na/gm	ANTIBIOTIC, penicillin **Drug:** Parenterally administered. **Diet:** Caution c̄ ↓ Na diet. **GI:** N&v, diarrhea. **S/Cond:** Caution c̄ lactation. **Metab/Phys:** Monitor electrolytes: possible hypokalemia in long term use.[3] **Other:** Altered taste. **Blood/Serum:** ↑ SGOT, ↑ SGPT, ↑ BUN, ↑ alk phos, ↑ creatinine, ↑ bilirubin, ↓ K. **Urinary:** false + protein.

MEDICATION	CLASSIFICATION & DIETARY/RELATED SIGNIFICANCES

miconazole nitrate
Monistat IV

ANTIFUNGAL
>**Drug:** Parenterally administered. **GI:** N&v, diarrhea.
>**Metab/Phys:** Monitor hematocrit, hemoglobin, electrolytes & lipids.
>**Other:** Drowsiness, anorexia.
>**Blood/Serum:** ↓ Na.

Micro-K

ELECTROLYTE

Contains 312mg K/cap.
See *potassium chloride.*

Micronase

ORAL HYPOGLYCEMIC

See *glyburide.*

Midol 200

ANTIARTHRITIC

See *ibuprofen.*

Milk of Magnesia
magnesium hydroxide
Suspension:
0.69mg Na/15ml

LAXATIVE, ANTACID
>**Drug:** Take c̄ fluids. Taste improved by following each dose c̄ citrus fruit juice. **Diet:** Encourage fluids unless otherwise directed.
>**Nutr:** Long term use: ↓ Thi, ↓ Ⓟ, ↓ Ca, ↓ Fe absorption.[11]
>**GI:** Belching, bloating, nausea. **Other:** Chalky taste.

Miltown

ANTIANXIETY

See *meprobamate.*

mineral oil **Agoral plain** **Mineral Oil**	LAXATIVE **Drug:** Take 2 hr away from food. Do not take at bedtime: possibility of oil aspiration causing lipid pneumonitis. **Nutr:** May ↓ absorption of Vit A, E, K. ↓ absorption of Vit D: impairs Ca & P absorption. **GI:** Indigestion, flatulence. **Other:** ↓ wt, anorexia.	
Minipress	ANTIHYPERTENSIVE	See *prazosin HCl.*
Minizide	ANTIHYPERTENSIVE c̄ DIURETIC	See *prazosin HCl.* See listing for *hydrochlorothiazide.*
minocycline HCl **Minocin**	ANTIBIOTIC, tetracycline **Drug:** May be taken c̄ food or milk. **Blood/Serum:** No BUN value.	See listing for *tetracycline.*
minoxidil **Loniten**	ANTIHYPERTENSIVE **Drug:** Take at same time each day. **Diet Important:** May need ↓ Na, ↓ cal diet. **S/Cond:** Caution c̄ lactation. **Metab/Phys:** Monitor fluid electrolytes & check body wt daily.[13] Edema. **Other:** Dizziness, headache. **Blood/Serum:** ↑ alk phos, ↑ creatinine, ↑ BUN, ↑ HCT, ↑ Hb (all transient), ↑ Na.[13]	
Mixtard	ANTIDIABETIC	See *insulin.*

See "Guide to the Use of This Book" p. 5 for explanation of format.

MEDICATION	CLASSIFICATION & DIETARY/RELATED SIGNIFICANCES	
Moduretic	ANTIHYPERTENSIVE c̄ DIURETIC	See *amiloride HCl.* See *hydrochlorothiazide.*
molindone HCl **Moban** 1.3gm sorbitol/5ml	ANTIPSYCHOTIC **Drug:** Take c̄ 8oz H_2O or milk to ↓ gastric irritation. **GI:** Constipation, nausea. **S/Cond:** Avoid alcohol. **Other:** <u>Drowsiness</u>, <u>dry mouth</u>, blurred vision, wt changes.	
Monistat IV	ANTIFUNGAL	See *miconazole nitrate.*
Monocid	ANTIBIOTIC	See *cefonicid Na.*
morphine sulfate **Morphine** Oral solution: lactose,[10] 10% alcohol[1]	ANALGESIC, NARCOTIC **Drug:** Parenterally & orally administered. **GI:** N&v, constipation. **S/Cond:** Not c̄ lactation. Avoid alcohol. **Metab/Phys:** Digestion of food delayed in small intestines. **Other:** <u>Drowsiness</u>, dry mouth, anorexia. **Blood/Serum:** ↑ amylase, ↑ lipase, ↓ lactate.	
Motrin	NSAI	See *ibuprofen.*
moxalactam **Moxam** 99mg Na/gm[7]	ANTIBIOTIC, cephalosporin **Drug:** Parenterally administered. **GI:** N&v. **S/Cond:** Avoid alcohol. **Metab/Phys:** Disulfiram like reaction. ↓ bacterial synthesis of Vit K	

in small intestines.
Blood/Serum: ↑ SGOT, ↑ SGPT, ↑ BUN, ↑ creatinine, ↑ alk phos.[3]

Mycelex-(Troche)	ANTIFUNGAL	See *clotrimazole*.
Mycifraden	ANTIBIOTIC	See *neomycin sulfate*.
Mycostatin	ANTIFUNGAL	Suspension: 2.5gm sucrose/5ml. See *nystatin*.

Mylanta
magnesium hydroxide, aluminum hydroxide & simethicone

ANTACID, ANTIFLATULENT
Drug: Chew tab. Take 1 hr after meals. 0.68mg Na/5ml, 0.77mg Na/tab. Liquid: 0.667gm sorbitol/5ml. **Nutr:** May ↓ absorption of Vit A. Long term use: ↓ P & Ca absorption. Inactivates Thi. **GI:** Constipation. **Metab/Phys:** Hypermagnesemia c̄ renal impairment.[4]

Mylanta II
magnesium & aluminum hydroxides, simethicone

ANTACID, ANTIFLATULENT

1.14mg Na/5ml.
1.3mg Na/tab.
Liquid: 0.667gm sorbitol/5ml.
See **Mylanta**.

Myleran   ANTINEOPLASTIC   See *busulfan*.

MEDICATION	CLASSIFICATION & DIETARY/RELATED SIGNIFICANCES

Mylicon ANTIFLATULENT See *simethicone.*

Mysoline ANTICONVULSANT See *primidone.*

Mysteclin F ANTIBIOTIC See *tetracycline HCl.*
tetracycline HCl & **Drug:** Contains 2.2gm sucrose/5ml, 21mg K/5ml. Cap contains lac-
amphotericin B tose. Syrup contains sulfites & 3mg Na/5ml. **Other:** Altered taste.

nadolol ANTIANGINAL, ANTIHYPERTENSIVE, beta blocker
Corgard **Drug:** May take $\bar{s}$ regard to meals.[7] **Diet Important:** Possible
↓ Na,[13] ↓ cal diet. Avoid natural licorice. **GI:** Constipation, GI
distress, nausea,[10] flatulence. **S/Cond:** Caution $\bar{c}$ diabetic: may
mask symptoms of hypoglycemia. **Other:** Dizziness, fatigue,
dry mouth.
Blood/Serum: ↑ K, ↓ HDL, ↑ TG, ↑ uric acid.

nafcillin Na ANTIBIOTIC
Nafcil **Drug:** Parenterally or orally administered. Take $\bar{c}$ 8oz H_2O
Unipen on empty stomach. Chew tab. **GI:** N&v, diarrhea.
67mg Na/gm **Metab/Phys:** Anemia.

Naldecon
 phenylpropanolamine,
 phenylephrine,
 phenyltoloxamine
 citrate & chlorphen-
 iramine maleate

DECONGESTANT
 Drug: Take c̄ food or H$_2$O. Pediatric syrup contains sorbitol, sucrose, 5% alcohol. **GI:** N&v. **S/Cond:** Caution c̄ diabetic: may ↑ blood glucose. **Other:** Drowsiness, dizziness, tremors, anorexia, blurred vision.[3]

Nalfon NSAI See *fenoprofen.*

nalidixic acid
 NegGram

ANTI-INFECTIVE, urinary
 Drug: Take c̄ 8oz of H$_2$O on empty stomach. If GI distress, take c̄ milk. **Diet:** Encourage ↑ fluids unless otherwise directed.
 GI: Diarrhea, n&v, abdominal pain. **Metab/Phys:** Blood dyscrasias.[13] **Other:** Blurred vision, colored vision changes, drowsiness, dizziness.[13]
 Urinary: ↑ glucose (c̄ CuSO$_4$).[3]

naltrexone
 Trexan

NARCOTIC DETERRENT
 GI: Abdominal pain, cramps, n&v. **Other:** Headache, tiredness.

See "Guide to the Use of This Book" p. 5 for explanation of format.

MEDICATION	CLASSIFICATION & DIETARY/RELATED SIGNIFICANCES
naproxen **Anaprox** 25mg Na/tab **Naprosyn**	ANTIARTHRITIC, NSAI, ANALGESIC **Drug:** Optimal: Take c̄ 8 oz H_2O.[13] **GI:** Constipation, dyspepsia, diarrhea, stomatitis, n&v, abdominal pain. **S/Cond:** Not c̄ lactation. Avoid alcohol. Diabetics: may have hypoglycemic effects. **Metab/Phys:** Edema. **Other:** ↑ wt, dizziness, drowsiness, visual problems. **Blood/Serum:** ↑ BUN, ↑ creatinine, ↑ K, ↑ SGOT, ↑ SGPT.
Nardil	ANTIDEPRESSANT See *phenelzine sulfate.*
Navane	ANTIPSYCHOTIC See *thiothixene.*
Nebcin	ANTIBIOTIC See *tobramycin sulfate.*
NegGram	ANTI-INFECTIVE See *nalidixic acid.*
Nembutal	SEDATIVE, HYPNOTIC See *pentobarbital.* Elixir: 18% alcohol; cap contains tartrazine.

neomycin sulfate   ANTIBIOTIC
Mycifraden
Neomycin Sulfate

    Diet: ↓ consumption of sweets. **Nutr:** Long term use: ↓ absorption of lipids, chol,[6] carotene, glucose, lactose, sucrose, Na, Ca, Fe, Vit A, D, K, B_{12}, Fol, & B_6. **GI:** N&v, diarrhea. **Metab/Phys:** Drug inhibits action of disaccharidose & lactose enzymes in intestines.[6] **Other:** Sore mouth.
    Blood/Serum: ↑ creatinine, ↑ BUN.
    Urinary: + protein.[3]

netilmicin sulfate   ANTIBIOTIC, aminoglycoside
Netromycin
Contains sulfites[7]

    Drug: Parenterally administered. **Diet:** Encourage ↑ fluids unless otherwise directed. **GI:** N&v, diarrhea. **Other:** Anorexia, ↑ thirst, dizziness.[13]
    Blood/Serum: ↑ BUN,[3] ↑ SGOT, ↑ SGPT, ↑ LDH, ↑ bilirubin, ↑ creatinine, ↓ Mg, ↓ Na, ↓ K, ↓ Ca, ↑ alk phos.
    Urinary: + for protein.

nicotine polacrilex   SMOKING DETERRENT
Nicorette
Sugar free

    Drug: Chew slowly. Loosens fillings in teeth.[13] **GI:** N&v, GI distress, belching, constipation. **Other:** Sore mouth & throat, hiccups, dizziness, ↑ salivation, ↑ appetite, headache.

MEDICATION	CLASSIFICATION & DIETARY/RELATED SIGNIFICANCES

nicotinic acid
Nicobid
Nico-400
Nicolar
Contains tartrazine

ANTIHYPERLIPEMIC
    Drug: Take $\bar{c}$ food. Swallow tab whole. **Diet:** Do not use vitamins as substitute for balanced diet. **GI:** N&v, bloating, cramps, diarrhea, flatulence. **S/Cond:** Monitor diabetic: ↓ glucose tolerance.[4]
    Metab/Phys: Hyperglycemia & hyperuricemia $\bar{c}$ large doses.
    Other: Dizziness.
    Blood/Serum: ↑ alk phos,[3] ↑ SGOT, ↑ SGPT, ↑ bilirubin, ↑ uric acid, ↑ glucose, ↓ LDH, ↑ HDL, ↓ albumin, ↓ chol, ↓ TG.
    Urinary: ↑ glucose (false + $\bar{c}$ $CuSO_4$).

nifedipine
Procardia

ANTIANGINAL, ANTIHYPERTENSIVE, Ca-channel blocker
    Drug: Take $\bar{c}$ food or milk.[13] **GI:** Nausea, diarrhea, constipation, cramps, flatulence. **S/Cond:** Monitor diabetic: May ↓ glucose tolerance. **Metab/Phys:** Edema. **Other:** Weakness, dizziness, headache, altered taste.[37].
    Blood/Serum: ↑ alk phos, ↑ SGOT, ↑ SGPT, ↑ LDH, ↑ CPK.

Nilstat

ANTIFUNGAL   70%/volume liquid glucose, sucrose.
                        See **nystatin.**

nitrofurantoin **Furadantin** Tab: sucrose, sorbitol **Macrodantin** Cap: lactose	ANTIBIOTIC, urinary **Drug:** Take $\bar{c}$ food or milk: food $\uparrow$ bioavailability. Liquid may be mixed $\bar{c}$ H_2O, milk or fruit juice. **Diet:** Monitor diet for adequacy in protein, B complex Vit.[1] **GI:** N&v, abdominal pain, diarrhea. **S/Cond:** Caution $\bar{c}$ lactation. **Metab/Phys:** Possible peripheral neuritis, hemolytic anemia $\bar{c}$ G6PD deficiency. **Other:** Anorexia, drowsiness, dizziness.[13] **Blood/Serum:** $\downarrow$ Fol.[11] **Urinary:** $\uparrow$ glucose (false + $\bar{c}$ $CuSO_4$).	
nitroglycerin **Nitrobid–injection** **Nitrodur–patch** **Nitrogard–buccal** **Nitrostat–sublingual** **Transderm-Nitro–patch**	ANTIANGINAL **Drug:** Consult Pharmacist or References 13, 7, or 10 for administration. **S/Cond:** Avoid alcohol. Caution $\bar{c}$ lactation. **GI:** Abdominal pain. **Other:** Dry mouth, headache, dizziness, blurred vision.	
Nizoral	ANTIFUNGAL	See *ketoconazole*.
Noctec	SEDATIVE	See *chloral hydrate*.
Nolvadex	ANTINEOPLASTIC	See *tamoxifen citrate*.

MEDICATION	CLASSIFICATION & DIETARY/RELATED SIGNIFICANCES

Nordette
*levonorgestrel &
ethinyl estradiol*

CONTRACEPTIVE, oral   See listing for *estrogens.*

*norethindrone
ethinyl estradiol*

CONTRACEPTIVE, oral   See listing for *estrogens.*

norfloxacin
Noroxin

ANTI-INFECTIVE, ANTIBIOTIC
    Drug: Take c̄ 8oz H_2O 1 hr before or 2 hr after meals.
    Diet: Maintain adequate fluid intake.[13]. **GI:** N&v, abdominal pain,
    heartburn, diarrhea. **S/Cond:** Not c̄ lactation. **Other:** Dizziness,
    headache, anorexia, sore mouth, ↓ salivation.
    Blood/Serum: ↑ SGOT, ↑ SGPT, ↑ alk phos, ↑ BUN, ↑ creati-
    nine, ↑ LDH, ↓ HCT.

Norgesic
*orphenadrine citrate
aspirin, caffeine*
30mg caffeine/tab
Norgesic forte
60mg caffeine/tab

MUSCLE RELAXANT, ANALGESIC
    Drug: Take c̄ food or 8oz H_2O. **GI:** N&v, constipation, heartburn.
    S/Cond: Avoid alcohol. **Other:** Drowsiness, blurred vision, dry
    mouth, confusion, especially in the elderly.
    Blood/Serum: ↑ or ↓ uric acid (dose related), ↓ T_4.
    Urinary: ↑ glucose (false + c̄ $CuSO_4$).

Norinyl *norethindrone c̄* *mestranol*	CONTRACEPTIVE	See listing for *estrogens*.
Normodyne	ANTIHYPERTENSIVE	See *labetalol HCl*.
Norpace	ANTIARRHYTHMIC	See *disopyramide phosphate*.
Norpramin	ANTIDEPRESSANT	See *desipramine HCl*.
nortriptyline HCl Aventyl Pamelor Solution: 4% alcohol	ANTIDEPRESSANT, tricyclic **DRUG:** Take c̄ food to ↓ gastric distress. **Diet:** ↑ need for Rib. **GI:** Epigastric distress, n&v, GI distress, diarrhea, constipation. **S/Cond:** Avoid alcohol. Caution c̄ lactation. **Metab/Phys:** Inappropriate ADH syndrome. Blood dyscrasias. **Other:** Peculiar taste, ↑ or ↓ wt, dry mouth, drowsiness, ↑ appetite for sweets, black tongue, dizziness, confusion, blurred vision. **Blood/Serum:** ↑ or ↓ glucose.	
Novafed Syrup: 7.5% alcohol	DECONGESTANT	See *pseudoephedrine HCl*.
Novolin	ANTIDIABETIC	See *insulin*.

MEDICATION	CLASSIFICATION & DIETARY/RELATED SIGNIFICANCES	
NPH Insulin *insulin, beef or pork*	ANTIDIABETIC	See *insulin.*
Numorphan	ANALGESIC	See *oxymorphone HCl.*
Nuprin	NSAI	See *ibuprofen.*
nystatin **Mycostatin** Oral suspension 1% alcohol, 50% sucrose **Nilstat**	ANTIFUNGAL	**Drug:** Take oral solution as directed. Retain drug in mouth as long as possible. Do not swallow lozenge whole. **GI:** Diarrhea, n&v, stomach pain.
Ogen	HORMONE	See listing for *estrogens.*
Omnipen *ampicillin*	ANTIBIOTIC, penicillin	See *ampicillin.*
Oncovin	ANTINEOPLASTIC	See *vincristine sulfate.*
Optimine	ANTIHISTAMINIC	Tab: lactose. See *azatadine maleate.*

Orasone *prednisone*	CORTICOSTEROID	See listing for ***hydrocortisone.***
Oretic	ANTIHYPERTENSIVE	See ***hydrochlorothiazide.***
Orinase	ORAL HYPOGLYCEMIC	See ***tolbutamide.***
Ornade *chlorpheniramine maleate,* *phenylpropanolamine HCl*	ANTIHISTAMINIC, DECONGESTANT **Drug:** Take c̄ food or H_2O. **GI:** N&v, GI distress, constipation. **S/Cond:** Avoid alcohol.[13] Monitor diabetic. **Metab/Phys:** Anemia. **Other:** Drowsiness, dizziness, dry mouth, anorexia.	
Orudis	ANTIARTHRITIC	See ***ketoprofen.***
Osmitrol	DIURETIC, DIAGNOSTIC	See ***mannitol.***
Ovral	CONTRACEPTIVE, oral	See listing for ***estrogens.***
Ovulen	CONTRACEPTIVE, oral	See listing for ***estrogens.***

MEDICATION	CLASSIFICATION & DIETARY/RELATED SIGNIFICANCES

oxacillin sodium
Powder for IV:
64mg Na/gm
Bactocill
Prostaphlin

ANTIBIOTIC, penicillin
Drug: Parenterally & orally administered. Oral: Take 1 hr before or 2 hr after meal. **Diet:** Acid stable. **GI:** Stomatitis, diarrhea, n&v, steatorrhea. **Metab/Phys:** Hypokalemia. **Other:** Glossitis, mouth sores/ulcers.
Blood/Serum: ↑ SGOT.

oxazepam
Serax
15mg tab:
tartrazine, lactose

ANTIANXIETY, benzodiazepine
Drug: May take c̄ food or H_2O. **GI:** Nausea. **S/Cond:** Avoid alcohol. **Metab/Phys:** Edema, blood dyscrasias. **Other:** Dizziness, drowsiness, tremors.

oxtriphylline
Choledyl
Elixir: 20% alcohol

BRONCHODILATOR
Drug: Optimal: Take on empty stomach to ↑ absorption. May take c̄ food. Swallow tab whole. **Diet:** Limit charcoal-broiled food. Avoid extremes of dietary protein & CHO.[14] **GI:** GI distress, n&v, diarrhea. **S/Cond:** Limit xanthine-containing foods or beverages: see Table p. 231.
Blood/Serum: ↑ glucose, ↑ uric acid, ↑ bilirubin.
Urinary: albumin.

oxybutynin chloride **Ditropan**	PARASYMPATHOLYTIC, ANTISPASMODIC, urinary **Drug:** Optimal: Take on empty stomach $\bar{c}$ 8oz H_2O. If GI upset may take $\bar{c}$ food or milk. **GI:** N&v, constipation. **S/Cond:** Avoid alcohol. Not $\bar{c}$ lactation. **Other:** Dry mouth, drowsiness, blurred vision, bloating, dizziness, fatigue.	
oxymorphone HCl **Numorphan**	ANALGESIC, NARCOTIC **Drug:** Administered parenterally or suppository. **GI:** Constipation, n&v. **S/Cond:** Avoid alcohol. **Other:** <u>Drowsiness</u>, dizziness, anorexia, dry mouth, headache. **Blood/Serum:** ↑ amylase, ↑ lipase.	
Pamelor	ANTIDEPRESSANT	See *nortriptyline.*
papaverine HCl **Pavabid**	CARDIOVASCULAR VASODILATOR **Drug:** Take $\bar{c}$ food. Swallow tab/cap whole. **GI:** Nausea, abdominal pain, diarrhea, constipation. **Other:** Dizziness, drowsiness, anorexia. **Blood/Serum:** ↑ alk phos, ↑ SGOT, ↑ SGPT.	
Paraflex	MUSCLE RELAXANT	See *chlorzoxazone.*
Parafon Forte	MUSCLE RELAXANT, ANALGESIC	See *chlorzoxazone.* See *acetaminophen.*

See "Guide to the Use of This Book" p. 5 for explanation of format.

MEDICATION	CLASSIFICATION & DIETARY/RELATED SIGNIFICANCES	
Paregoric *camphorated* *tincture of opium* 45% alcohol	ANTIDIARRHEAL, NARCOTIC **Drug:** May take c̄ food. **GI:** N&v, constipation, **S/Cond:** Avoid alcohol. **Metab/Phys:** Fluid loss. **Other:** Dizziness, drowsiness.	
Parlodel	ANTIPARKINSONISM	See *bromocriptine.*
Parnate	ANTIDEPRESSANT, MAOI	See *tranylcypromine sulfate.*
P.A.S. *aminosalicylate Na*	ANTITUBERCULAR	See *aminosalicylate Na.*
Pathocil	ANTIBIOTIC, penicillin	See *dicloxacillin sodium.*
Pavabid	VASODILATOR	See *papaverine HCl.*
Pediamycin *erythromycin* *ethylsuccinate*	ANTIBIOTIC	See *erythromycin.*

Pediazole
erythromycin ethylsuccinate & sulfisoxazole acetyl

ANTIBIOTIC, sulfonamide
Drug: Take s̄ regard to meals. **Diet:** Most soluble in alkaline urine.[1] Encourage ↑ fluids unless otherwise directed. **GI:** N&v, diarrhea, GI distress, cramps. **S/Cond:** Not c̄ lactation. **Metab/Phys:** Caution c̄ G6PD deficiency. Possible hypoglycemia, hepatitis.
Other: Dizziness, anorexia.
Blood/Serum: ↑ alk phos, ↑ bilirubin, ↑ SGOT, ↑ SGPT, ↓ glucose (rare).
Urinary: ↑ glucose (false + $CuSO_4$), + protein.

penicillamine
Cuprimine
Depen

ANTIARTHRITIC, HEAVY METAL ANTAGONIST
Drug: Take 2 hr before or 2 hr after meals. (Infants, children: dissolve in juice). Rheumatoid Arthritis: Take on an empty stomach, 1 hr apart from any food, meals, milk or snacks. **Diet:** For Wilson's disease: ↓ Cu diet (less than 1–2mg Cu daily) omit chocolate, nuts, shellfish, mushrooms, liver, raisins, molasses, broccoli, cereal ↑ in Cu. Use distilled H_2O if local H_2O contains more than 0.1mg Cu/L. Lead poisoning: ↓ Ca diet. Kidney stones: ↑ fluid intake & keep urine alkaline (pH 7.5), ↓ methionine diet (modified Giovannetti), except children & in pregnancy. Supplements: Fe & Zn may interfere c̄ drug action. **Nutr:** ↑ requirement for Pyr; ↑ excretion of Zn, Fe, Cu, & Pyr. Possible Fe deficiency & anemias. Pyr may correct drug-induced peripheral neuropathy.[14] **GI:** N&v, diarrhea.
Other: ↓ taste for salt & sweet, anorexia, unpleasant taste.
Blood/Serum: ↑ alk phos, ↑ LDH.
Urinary: ↑ Cu, ↑ Zn.

See "Guide to the Use of This Book" p. 5 for explanation of format.

MEDICATION	CLASSIFICATION & DIETARY/RELATED SIGNIFICANCES

penicillin

ANTIBIOTIC
Drug: Take c̄ 8oz H$_2$O on empty stomach. **GI:** N&v, diarrhea, gastritis, flatulence. **S/Cond:** Anemias. **Other:** Black, hairy tongue, sore mouth, altered taste (may ↓ appetite).

Bicillin: 10mg Na/5ml suspension.
Penicillin G Buffered: 39mg Na/5 million units.
Penicillin G Potassium: 69mg Na/1 million units; 16.40mg K/250,000 units; 2.7gm sucrose/5ml.[29]
Penicillin G Sodium: 46mg Na/1 million units.
Pentids: 2.8gm sucrose/5ml; 20 Na/200,000 units/5ml; tartrazine.

penicillin V potassium
Betapen VK

ANTIBIOTIC   See **penicillin.**

Ledercillin 125mg sucrose/5ml.
Pen Vee K 38mg Na/250mg, 28.8mg K.

pentaerythritol tetranitrate
Peritrate

ANTIANGINAL
Drug: Take c̄ 8oz H$_2$O on empty stomach. Do not crush or chew sustained released caps: Swallow whole. **GI;** N&v, GI distress, **S/Cond:** Avoid alcohol. **Other:** Headache, dizziness.

pentazocine HCl **Talwin NX**	ANALGESIC	**GI:** N&v, GI distress. **S/Cond:** Avoid alcohol. **Other:** Drowsiness, dizziness, anorexia, dry mouth, altered taste.[3] **Blood/Serum:** ↑ amylase, ↑ lipase.
pentobarbital **Nembutal** Elixir: 18% alcohol[3] 100mg cap: tartrazine 50mg cap: lactose[10]	SEDATIVE, HYPNOTIC	**Drug:** Take c̄ H$_2$O, milk, or juice. **Diet:** Supplements: Pyr ↓ drug effects.[9] **S/Cond:** Avoid alcohol. Not c̄ lactation. **Other:** Drowsiness, dizziness. Chronic use: ↓ appetite, ↓ wt. **Blood/Serum:** ↓ bilirubin.
pentoxifylline **Trental**	HEMORRHEOLOGIC	**Drug:** Take c̄ meals or food.[13] **Diet Important:** ↓ cal, ↓ chol diet may be recommended.[17] **GI:** N&v, dyspepsia, belching, diarrhea, abdominal pain, constipation, flatulence. **S/Cond:** Not c̄ lactation. **Metab/Phys:** Edema. **Other:** Dizziness, headache, anorexia, dry mouth, sore throat, thirst, blurred vision.
Pepcid	ANTIULCER	See *famotidine*.
Pepto-Bismol	ANTIDIARRHEAL	See *bismuth subsalicylate*.

See "Guide to the Use of This Book" p. 5 for explanation of format.

MEDICATION	CLASSIFICATION & DIETARY/RELATED SIGNIFICANCES

Percocet-5
oxycodone HCl &
acetaminophen

ANALGESIC, NARCOTIC
    GI: N&v, constipation. **S/Cond:** Avoid alcohol. **Other:** Dizziness,
sedation, ↓ appetite, dry mouth.
    Blood/Serum: ↑ amylase, ↑ lipase.

Percodan
oxycodone HCl,
aspirin, & oxycodone
terephthalate

ANALGESIC, NARCOTIC
    Drug: Take c̄ food or 8oz H$_2$O. **GI:** N&v, constipation.
    S/Cond: Avoid alcohol. **Other:** Dizziness, dry mouth.
    Blood/Serum: ↑ lipase, ↑ amylase, ↓ T$_4$, ↑ or ↓ uric acid,
dose-related.
    Urinary: ↑ glucose (false + c̄ CuSO$_4$).

Perdiem, plain   LAXATIVE   See *psyllium.*

Periactin   ANTIHISTAMINIC   See *cyproheptadine HCl.*

Peritrate   ANTIANGINAL   See *pentaerythritol tetranitrate.*

perphenazine **Trilafon**	ANTIPSYCHOTIC, ANTINAUSEANT **Drug:** Take c̄ food. Swallow tab whole. Do not dilute concentrate c̄ caffeine, tannics (tea) or pectinates (apple juice) containing beverages. See Table p. 231. **GI:** Constipation. **S/Cond:** Avoid alcohol. Monitor diabetic. **Metab/Phys:** Hypo/hyperglycemia, jaundice, edema. **Other:** Drowsiness, dry mouth, anorexia, blurred vision, dizziness. **Blood/Serum:** ↑ glucose. **Urinary:** ↑ bilirubin (false elevation).	
Persantine	ANTIPLATELET	See *dipyridamole*.
Pertofrane	ANTIDEPRESSANT	See *desipramine HCl*.
Phenaphen c̄ Codeine	ANALGESIC, NARCOTIC	See *acetaminophen*. See *codeine*.
phenazopyridine HCl **Pyridium**	ANALGESIC, urinary **Drug:** Take c̄ food. **GI:** GI distress. **S/Cond:** Monitor diabetic: false urinary glucose & ketone test.[13] **Metab/Phys:** Anemia. **Other:** Headache.	

See "Guide to the Use of This Book" p. 5 for explanation of format.

168

| MEDICATION | CLASSIFICATION & DIETARY/RELATED SIGNIFICANCES |

MEDICATION

CLASSIFICATION & DIETARY/RELATED SIGNIFICANCES

phenelzine sulfate
Nardil

ANTIDEPRESSANT, MAOI
    Diet Important: Avoid foods ↑ in pressor amines. See Table
p. 234. Limit caffeine-containing foods & beverages.[14] See Table
p. 231. Supplements: Tryptophan may result in headache, hypertension.[14] **GI:** Constipation, GI distress. **S/Cond:** Avoid alcohol.
Monitor diabetic: hypoglycemic effect may be ↑ .
    Metab/Phys: Edema. Possible fluid & electrolyte imbalance.[10]
    Other: Dizziness, drowsiness, ↑ or ↓ wt, tremors, dry mouth,
blurred vision,[7] hyperexcitability.[7]
    Blood/Serum: ↓ glucose.[3]

Phenergan

ANTIHISTAMINIC   See ***promethazine HCl.***

phenmetrazine HCl
Preludin
  75mg sustained
  release tab:
    tartrazine

APPETITE SUPPRESSANT
    Drug: Swallow whole. Take extended release tab 10–14 hr before
bedtime. Regular form: 4–6 hr before bedtime. **GI:** Constipation.
    S/Cond: Avoid alcohol. Monitor diabetic: may ↓ blood glucose.
    Other: Dizziness, drowsiness, dry mouth, unpleasant taste,[10]
blurred vision.

phenobarbital
Phenobarbital
Elixir: 0.635gm
sucrose/5ml

SEDATIVE, HYPNOTIC, ANTICONVULSANT
Drug: Take liquid $\bar{c}$ H$_2$O, milk, or juices. **Diet:** Vit doses (80–400mg) Pyr may ↓ drug effects.[14] **Nutr:** ↓ serum levels $\bar{c}$ Vit B$_{12}$, Fol, Ca, Mg, Pyr.[11] **GI:** N&v, diarrhea, epigastric pain. **S/Cond:** Caution $\bar{c}$ lactation. Avoid alcohol. **Metab/Phys:** ↑ catabolism of Vit K,[11] ↓ bone density, osteomalacia, ↑ turnover of Vit D & K, especially in children, possible neonatal hemmorhaging. **Other:** Dizziness, headache, confusion.
Blood/Serum: ↓ bilirubin.

phenolphthalein
Correctol
7.8mg Na/100mg tab
Ex-lax
0.53mg Na/tab

CATHARTIC
Drug: Take on empty stomach $\bar{c}$ 8oz H$_2$O. Chew tab/wafer well. Encourage ↑ fluids unless otherwise directed.[14]
Nutr: ↓ absorption of Vit D & C. **GI:** Steatorrhea.[11]
Metab/Phys: Prolonged use: electrolyte imbalance. Osteomalacia, hypokalemia.

phentermine HCl
Fastin
phentermine resin
Ionamin
Contains lactose[13]

APPETITE SUPPRESSANT
Drug: Swallow cap/tab whole. Take ½ hr before meals. May mask taste $\bar{c}$ fruit juice. **GI:** GI distress, constipation. **S/Cond:** Limit caffeine: see Table p. 231. Monitor diabetic: insulin effects may be altered.[10] Avoid alcohol. **Other:** Dizziness, tremors, dry mouth, unpleasant taste.

MEDICATION	CLASSIFICATION & DIETARY/RELATED SIGNIFICANCES

phenylbutazone
  Azolid
  Butazolidin

NSAI, ANTIGOUT, ANTIARTHRITIC
  Drug: Take c̄ 8oz H_2O, food or milk. **Nutr:** ↓ absorption of Fol, tryptophan, amino acids.[11] **Diet:** A Na restricted diet may be advised.[15] **GI:** Nausea, dyscrasias, GI distress, heartburn, constipation. **S/Cond:** Not c̄ lactation. Avoid alcohol.
  Metab/Phys: Hyperglycemia, ↑ or ↓ thyroid activity, blood dyscrasias, edema. **Other:** Drowsiness, headache, altered taste,[29] ↑ wt.

phenylpropanolamine
  Acutrim
  Control
  Dexatrim
  Prolamine

APPETITE SUPPRESSANT, DECONGESTANT
  Drug: Swallow tab/cap whole several hr before bedtime. **Diet Important:** ↓ cal for best effect. **GI:** N&v, stomach pain. **S/Cond:** Caution c̄ diabetic. Limit caffeine-containing beverages: see Table p. 231.
  Other: Drowsiness, dry mouth, headache.

phenytoin sodium
  Dilantin
  Cap: 8mg Na/100mg
  Liquid: 0.6% alcohol
  Extended release cap:
    lactose/sucrose

ANTICONVULSANT
  Drug: Take c̄ food or milk. Swallow extended release cap whole. Crush or chew chewables. **Diet:** Caution c̄ Ca, Pyr, & Fol supplements: Ca ↓ bioavailability of both drug & mineral; Pyr may ↓ drug effects; Fol may alter drug response. Avoid large intake of fluids.[14] Monitor weight. **Nutr:** Tube feedings ↓ bioavailability of drug. Monitor closely. ↑ turnover of Vit D & K, especially in children.[11] May cause rickets or osteomalacia. **GI:** N&v, constipation. **S/Cond:** Avoid

alcohol. Monitor diabetic: hyperglycemia. **Metab/Phys:** Anemia.[1]
Other: Altered taste, gum hypertrophy, drowsiness, dizziness, confusion.
Blood/Serum: ↓ Fol, ↓ Vit B_{12}, ↓ Pyr, ↓ Vit D, ↓ Ca, ↓ Mg, ↑ Cu, ↑ glucose, ↑ alk phos, ↑ GGT.

pilocarpine HCl
Isopto-Carpine

OPHTHALMIC for glaucoma
    GI: N&v, diarrhea, abdominal pain. **Other:** Tremors, ↑ salivation.

pindolol
Visken

ANTIHYPERTENSIVE, beta blocker
    Drug: Take s̄ regard to meals.[7] **GI:** Diarrhea, vomiting. **S/Cond:** Limit alcohol. Not c̄ lactation. Monitor diabetic: may mask symptoms of hypoglycemia. May alter glucose tolerance.[13] **Metab/Phys:** Edema.
Other: Dizziness, fatigue.
Blood/Serum: ↑ SGOT, ↑ SGPT, ↓ HDL, ↑ TG, ↑ BUN, ↑ uric acid, ↑ K.[1]

piperacillin sodium
Pipracil
42mg Na/gm

ANTIBIOTIC, penicillin
    Drug: Parenterally administered. **GI:** Diarrhea, n&v, stomach pain. **S/Cond:** Caution c̄ lactation. **Metab/Phys:** Monitor electrolytes.
Other: Headache, fatigue.
Blood/Serum: ↑ BUN, ↑ creatinine, ↑ SGOT, ↑ SGPT, ↑ LDH, ↓ K.

MEDICATION	CLASSIFICATION & DIETARY/RELATED SIGNIFICANCES	
piroxicam **Feldene**	NSAI **Drug:** Take c̄ food. **GI:** <u>Epigastric distress</u>, nausea, constipation, diarrhea, flatulence. **S/Cond:** Not c̄ lactation. **Metab/Phys:** <u>Edema</u>. **Other:** <u>Dizziness</u>, anorexia, headache. **Blood/Serum:** ↑ BUN, ↓ HCT, ↓ Hb, ↑ SGOT, ↑ SGPT, ↑ creatinine. **Urinary:** + protein.	
Placidyl	HYPNOTIC	See *ethchlorvynol.*
Platinol	ANTINEOPLASTIC	See *cisplatin.*
Polaramine	ANTIHISTAMINIC	See *dexchlorpheniramine maleate.*
Polycillin	ANTIBIOTIC	See *ampicillin.*
Polymox	ANTIBIOTIC	See *amoxicillin.*
polythiazide **Renese**	ANTIHYPERTENSIVE, DIURETIC	See listing for *hydrochlorothiazide.*
Pondimin	APPETITE SUPPRESSANT	See *fenfluramine HCl.*

Ponstel	ANALGESIC	See ***mefenamic acid.***

potassium acid phosphate
K-Phos Original
114mg P,
144mg K/tab
Na free

ACIDIFIER, PHOSPHORUS PREPARATION
Drug: Take $\bar{c}$ 8oz H_2O after meals, or $\bar{c}$ food to ↓ GI upset. Swallow cap whole. **Diet:** Encourage ↑ fluids unless otherwise directed. **GI:** N&v, diarrhea, abdominal pain. **Metab/Phys:** Monitor electrolytes. ↑ wt (pedal edema). **Other:** Dizziness, ↑ thirst, fatigue.
Blood/Serum: ↓ Ca, ↑ P.[7]
Urinary: ↓ Ca.[1]

potassium chloride
Kaochlor, et al
Micro-K
Slow-K

ELECTROLYTE
Drug: Give $\bar{c}$ food. Liquid & soluble granules: dilute or dissolve in H_2O or juice (juice masks bitter taste). Swallow enteric-coated tab/cap whole. **Diet:** No ↑ Na juices or salt substitutes.[13]
Nutr: Malabsorption of B_{12}. **GI:** N&v, diarrhea, GI distress.
S/Cond: Caution $\bar{c}$ lactation. **Metab/Phys:** Possible hyperkalemia.
Other: Confusion, weakness.
Blood/Serum: ↑ K.
Urinary: ↑ K.

MEDICATION	CLASSIFICATION & DIETARY/RELATED SIGNIFICANCES
prazepam **Centrax**	ANTIANXIETY, benzodiazepine **GI:** Diarrhea. **S/Cond:** Not c̄ lactation. Avoid alcohol. Limit caffeine: see Table p. 231. **Other:** <u>Fatigue</u>, <u>dizziness</u>, <u>drowsiness</u>, <u>weakness</u>, blurred vision, tremors, ↑ appetite, ↑ wt, dry mouth, confusion. **Blood/Serum:** albumin.
prazosin HCl **Minipress**	ANTIHYPERTENSIVE **Diet Important:** Possible ↓ cal, ↓ Na diet. **GI:** Nausea, diarrhea, constipation, GI distress. **S/Cond:** Limit alcohol. **Metab/Phys:** <u>Edema</u>. **Other:** <u>Dizziness</u>, <u>drowsiness</u>, <u>dry mouth</u>, <u>weakness</u>, <u>headache</u>, blurred vision.[3]
Precef	ANTIBIOTIC — See *ceforanide.*
prednisolone **Prednisolone**	CORTICOSTEROID — See listing for *hydrocortisone.*
prednisone **Deltasone** **Orasone** **Prednisone**	CORTICOSTEROID — See listing for *hydrocortisone.*

Preludin	APPETITE SUPPRESSANT	See ***phenmetrazine HCl.***
Premarin *conjugated estrogen*	HORMONE	See ***estrogens.***
Primaxin	ANTIBIOTIC	See ***imipenem*** & ***cilastatin.***

primidone
  Mysoline
    ANTICONVULSANT
        Drug: Take c̄ food. **Diet:** Encourage foods ↑ in Vit K, C, D, & B$_{12}$.
        Nutr: ↑ turnover of Vit D & K, especially in children; osteomalacia. ↓ Ca absorption,[29] may impair Fol metabolism. **GI:** N&v.
        S/Cond: Not c̄ lactation. Avoid alcohol. **Metab/Phys:** Megaloblastic anemia. **Other:** Anorexia, fatigue, drowsiness, dizziness, headache.
        Blood/Serum: ↓ Fol, ↓ Vit B$_{12}$, ↓ Pyr, ↓ bilirubin.

Principen *ampicillin trihydrate*	ANTIBIOTIC Suspension: 250mg Na/5ml; 3.2gm sucrose/5ml. Cap: lactose.	See ***ampicillin.***
Prinivil	ANTIHYPERTENSIVE	See ***lisinopril.***
Pro-Banthine	ANTISPASMODIC	See ***propantheline bromide.***

MEDICATION	CLASSIFICATION & DIETARY/RELATED SIGNIFICANCES

probenecid
Benemid

ANTIGOUT, uricosuric
> **Drug:** Take c̄ food to ↓ gastric irritation. **Diet:** Encourage ↑ fluids unless otherwise directed. More effective in alkaline urine.[10] See Table p. 238. **Nutr:** ↓ absorption of Rib & amino acids.[11] **GI:** N&v. **S/Cond:** Avoid alcohol. **Other:** Anorexia, sore gums, dizziness, headache.
> **Blood/Serum:** ↓ uric acid.
> **Urinary:** ↑ uric acid, ↑ Rib, ↑ Ca, ↑ Mg, ↑ Na, ↑ K, ↑ Cl, ↓ pantothenic acid, ↑ glucose (false + c̄ $CuSO_4$).

probucol
Lorelco

ANTIHYPERLIPEMIC
> **Drug:** Take c̄ food to maximize absorption. **Diet:** Follow prescribed diet. **GI:** N&v, flatulence, diarrhea. **S/Cond:** Not c̄ lactation. Avoid alcohol. Monitor diabetic. **Other:** Bloating, anorexia, altered taste/smell, dizziness, headache.
> **Blood/Serum:** ↑ alk phos, ↑ BUN, ↑ SGOT, ↑ SGPT, ↑ bilirubin, ↑ glucose, ↑ uric acid, ↑ CPK, ↓ Hb, ↓ HCT.

procainamide HCl
  Procan SR
  Pronestyl
  250 & 375 tab: tartrazine
  Cap (except 500mg): lactose
  Vials: sulfites

ANTIARRHYTHMIC
  Drug: Take c̄ 8oz H$_2$O on empty stomach. Swallow sustained release tab whole. **GI:** Diarrhea, n&v. **S/Cond:** Not c̄ lactation. **Metab/Phys:** Agranulocytosis. **Other:** Anorexia, giddiness, bitter taste, sore mouth.
  Blood/Serum: ↑ SGOT, ↑ SGPT, ↑ alk phos, ↑ LDH, ↑ bilirubin.[13]

procarbazine HCl
  Matulane

ANTINEOPLASTIC
  Drug: Take c̄ food to ↓ n&v. **Diet Important:** Avoid foods high in pressor amines or caffeine. See Tables pp. 231 & 234. **GI:** N&v, stomatitis, constipation. **S/Cond:** Avoid alcohol: disulfiram-like reaction. Monitor diabetic: may alter insulin requirements.[13] Exhibits some MAOI activity.[11] **Metab/Phys:** Anemia. **Other:** Sore throat, dry mouth, anorexia, headache.

Procardia   ANTIANGINAL   See *nifedipine.*

MEDICATION	CLASSIFICATION & DIETARY/RELATED SIGNIFICANCES

prochlorperazine
Compazine
Ampule: sulfites
Tab/cap: sucrose

ANTIEMETIC, ANTIPSYCHOTIC
Drug: Take c̄ food or 8oz H_2O. Swallow extended release cap whole. **Diet:** ↑ need for Rib.[13] **GI:** Constipation. **S/Cond:** Not c̄ lactation. Avoid alcohol. Limit caffeine: see Table p. 231. Monitor diabetic. **Metab/Phys:** Anemias, edemas. **Other:** Dry mouth, blurred vision, drowsiness, ↑ wt, ↑ appetite.
Blood/Serum: ↑ SGOT, ↑ SGPT, ↑ LDH, ↑ alk phos, ↑ or ↓ glucose.

Progestin

ANTINEOPLASTIC

See **megestrol acetate.**

Prolamine

APPETITE SUPPRESSANT

See **phenylpropranalamine.**

Prolixin

ANTIPSYCHOTIC

See **fluphenazine HCl.**

Proloid
thyroglobulin

THYROID PREPARATION

See listing for **thyroid.**

promethazine HCl
Phenergan
Syrup: 7% alcohol[7]
Expectorant: 2.75ml
glucose/5ml[32]

ANTIHISTAMINIC, ANITVERTIGO, ANTIEMETIC
Drug: Take c̄ meals or 8oz H_2O or milk to ↓ gastric irritation.
Diet: ↑ need for Rib. **GI:** N&v. **S/Cond:** Caution c̄ lactation. Avoid alcohol. **Other:** Drowsiness, blurred vision, dry mouth, dizziness, confusion, taste changes.

57mg Na 7.1mg K/5ml	**Blood/Serum:** ↑ glucose.[3]	
promethazine HCl c̄ *codeine*	ANTIHISTAMINIC	See *codeine*. See *promethazine HCl*.
	Blood/Serum: ↑ lipase, ↑ amylase, ↑ glucose.	
Pronestyl	ANTIARRHYTHMIC	See *procainamide HCl*.

propantheline bromide
Pro-Banthine

ANTISPASMODIC, ANTICHOLINERGIC
Drug: Take ½ hr before meals. **GI:** Constipation, ↓ gastric emptying. **S/Cond:** Limit alcohol. Caution c̄ lactation. **Other:** Dry mouth, altered taste, confusion, dizziness, drowsiness, bloating, blurred vision.

propoxyphene HCl
Darvon
 Suspension: 2.5mg
  sucrose/5ml
Dolene

ANALGESIC
Drug: Take c̄ 8oz H$_2$O on empty stomach. May be taken c̄ food to prevent irritation. **GI:** N&v, constipation. **S/Cond:** Avoid alcohol. **Other:** Dizziness, drowsiness, light headedness, ↓ appetite, headache, weakness.
Blood/Serum: ↑ amylase, ↑ lipase, ↑ SGOT, ↑ SGPT, ↑ alk phos, ↑ LDH, ↑ bilirubin,[13] ↑ uric acid.

See "Guide to the Use of This Book" p. 5 for explanation of format.

MEDICATION	CLASSIFICATION & DIETARY/RELATED SIGNIFICANCES

propranolol HCl
Inderal

ANTIARRHYTHMIC, ANTIHYPERTENSIVE, beta blocker, ANTIMIGRAINE
Drug: Take c̄ food, enhances absorption.[7] **Diet Important:** Possible ↓ Na, ↓ cal diet. Avoid natural licorice. **GI:** Constipation, GI distress, nausea. **S/Cond:** Caution c̄ lactation. Limit alcohol. Monitor diabetic: may mask symptoms of hypoglycemia. **Other:** Dizziness, fatigue, dry mouth.
Blood/Serum: ↓ glucose, ↓ HDL, ↑ TG, ↑ BUN, ↑ uric acid, ↑ SGOT, ↑ SGPT, ↑ alk phos, ↑ LDH, ↑ T_4, ↓ T_3, ↑ K.[13]

propylthiouracil
Propyl-Thyracil (PTU)

ANTITHYROID
Drug: Take c̄ food same time each day. **GI:** N&v, epigastric distress. **S/Cond:** Not c̄ lactation. **Metab/Phys:** Edema. **Other:** Altered taste, dizziness.
Blood/Serum: ↑ LDH, ↑ SGPT, ↑ SGOT, ↑ alk phos, ↑ bilirubin.

Prostaphlin

ANTIBIOTIC, penicillin   See **_oxacillin sodium._**
Cap: 15mg Na/250mg. IV: 64mg Na/gm.

protriptyline HCl **Vivactil**	ANTIDEPRESSANT, tricyclic	

    Drug: May take c̄ food to ↓ GI upset. **Diet:** ↑ need for Rib.
    GI: Constipation, abdominal cramps, stomatitis, diarrhea.
    S/Cond: Avoid alcohol. Monitor diabetic. Limit caffeine: see Table p. 231. **Metab/Phys:** Blood dyscrasias. Inappropriate ADH syndrome. **Other:** Dry mouth, dizziness, ↑ or ↓ wt, blurred vision, confusion, especially in the elderly, ↑ appetite for sweets, altered taste, headache.
    Blood/Serum: ↑ or ↓ glucose.

Proventil	BRONCHODILATOR	See ***albuterol sulfate***.
Provera	HORMONE	See ***medroxyprogesterone acetate***.
Prozac	ANTIDEPRESSANT	See ***fluoxetine***.
pseudoephedrine HCl **Novafed** **Sudafed** Syrup: 2.4% alcohol	DECONGESTANT	

    Drug: Take c̄ H_2O or milk to ↓ GI irritation. Take last dose a few hr before bedtime. Swallow tab whole. Cap: Contents may be mixed c̄ jam or jelly. **GI:** Nausea. **S/Cond:** Not c̄ lactation. Caution c̄ diabetic. **Other:** Dizziness, tremors, headache, dry mouth.

MEDICATION

CLASSIFICATION & DIETARY/RELATED SIGNIFICANCES

psyllium hydrophilic mucilloid
  Fiberall
  Powder: 10mg Na,
    60mg K, 6 cal/dose
  Metamucil
  Powder: 1mg Na,
    31mg K,
    14 cal/dose
  Perdiem
  Plain: 2mg Na,
    35mg K/tsp

LAXATIVE, bulk-forming
  Drug: Take c̅ large amounts of fluids. **Diet:** Appropriate for ↓ Na diet. ↓ Rib absorption.[11] **GI:** Flatulence, n&v, steatorrhea, diarrhea. **Metab/Phys:** Long term use alters transport of electrolytes & ↓ plasma chol.

Purinethol	ANTINEOPLASTIC	See *mercaptopurine.*
Pyopen	ANTIBIOTIC	See *carbenicillin disodium.*
Pyridium	ANALGESIC	See *phenazopyridine HCl.*
PZI Iletin *protamine zinc insulin*	ANTIDIABETIC	See **Insulin.**

Questran *cholestyramine*	ANTIHYPERLIPEMIC	3.79gm sucrose/9gm packet. See ***cholestyramine***.
Quibron *theophylline &* *guaifenesin*	BRONCHODILATOR	See listing for ***theophylline***. See listing for ***guaifenesin***.

quinidine gluconate
   Quinaglute
      ANTIARRHYTHMIC
      Drug: Take c̄ 8oz H$_2$O on empty stomach. If GI distress, take c̄ food or milk. Swallow tab whole. **Diet:** <u>Avoid excessive intake of citrus juices; i.e. orange, grapefruit, pineapple and grape juice.[5] May ↑ need for Vit K.</u>[13] **GI:** N&v, diarrhea, stomach pain. **S/Cond:** Not c̄ lactation. **Metab/Phys:** Anemias.[3] **Other:** Bitter taste, anorexia, dizziness, visual problems, headache.

quinidine sulfate	ANTIARRHYTHMIC	See listing for ***quinidine gluconate***.

quinine sulfate
   Quinamm
   Quinine
      MUSCLE RELAXANT, ANTIMALARIAL
      Drug: Take c̄ food. **Diet:** May ↑ need for Vit K.[13] **GI:** GI distress, diarrhea. **Metab/Phys:** Blood dyscrasias. **Other:** Blurred vision, headache.

MEDICATION	CLASSIFICATION & DIETARY/RELATED SIGNIFICANCES

ranitidine
Zantac

ANTISECRETORY, ANTIULCER
 Nutr: ↓ Vit B_{12} in long term care. **GI:** Nausea, constipation, abdominal pain. **Other:** Headache, dizziness.
 Blood/Serum: ↑ SGOT, ↑ SGPT, ↑ GGT, ↑ creatinine.
 Urinary: + protein.

rauwolfia serpentina
Raudixin
Contains tartrazine, lactose, sucrose

ANTIHYPERTENSIVE
 Drug: Take c̄ food or milk to ↓ GI irritation.[13] **Diet Important:** ↓ Na, ↓ cal diet may be recommended. **GI:** Diarrhea, n&v. ↑ GI motility & gastric acid secretion. **S/Cond:** Not c̄ lactation. Avoid alcohol. Monitor diabetic: ↓ CHO tolerance.
 Metab/Phys: Na & H_2O retention.[1] **Other:** Anorexia, ↑ wt, drowsiness, lethargy, depression, dry mouth.

Rauzide

ANTIHYPERTENSIVE c̄ DIURETIC
 See **rauwolfia serpentina.** See listing for **hydrochlorothiazide.**

Reglan

GI STIMULANT   See **metoclopramide HCl.**

Regroton

ANTIHYPERTENSIVE   See listing for **rauwolfia serpentina.**
          See **chlorthalidone.**

Regular Insulin *insulin, beef & pork*	ANTIDIABETIC	See *insulin*.
Rela	MUSCLE RELAXANT	See *carisoprodol*.
Renese	ANTIHYPERTENSIVE	See listing for *hydrochlorothiazide*.
reserpine **Serpasil**	ANTIHYPERTENSIVE	See listing for *rauwolfia serpentina*.
Restoril	HYPNOTIC	See *temazepam*.
Retrovir	ANTIVIRAL	See *zidovudine*.
ribavirin **Tribavirin** **Virazole**	ANTIVIRAL	**S/Cond:** Not c̄ lactation. **Metab/Phys:** Anemia. **Other:** Blurred vision, dizziness. **Blood/Serum:** ↓ Hb, ↑ bilirubin.
ricinus communis	CATHARTIC	See *Castor Oil*.

See "Guide to the Use of This Book" p. 5 for explanation of format.

MEDICATION	CLASSIFICATION & DIETARY/RELATED SIGNIFICANCES
rifampin **Rifadin**	ANTIBIOTIC, ANTITUBERCULAR **Drug:** Take $\bar{c}$ 8oz H_2O on empty stomach. For children, mix cap $\bar{c}$ applesauce or jelly.[13] **GI:** Epigastric distress, cramps, diarrhea. **S/Cond:** Avoid alcohol. May interfere $\bar{c}$ serum folate and B_{12} tests.[10] **Other:** Red/orange colored saliva, anorexia, dizziness, confusion, altered taste.[38] **Blood/Serum:** ↑ SGOT, ↑ alk phos, ↑ BUN, ↑ bilirubin, ↑ uric acid.
Riopan *magaldrate* **Riopan Plus** *magaldrate &* *simethicone*	ANTACID, ANTIFLATULENT **Drug:** Take on empty stomach. ↓ than 0.1mg Na/tab. **Diet:** Useful $\bar{c}$ ↓ Na diet. **Nutr:** ↓ absorption of fat soluble vitamins, especially Vit A. **Other:** Chalky taste.
Ritalin	PSYCHOSTIMULANT See *methylphenidate HCl.*
Robaxin	MUSCLE RELAXANT See *methocarbamol.*
Rocephin	ANTIBIOTIC See *ceftriaxone.*
Rolaids	ANTACID See *dihydroxyaluminum sodium carbonate.*

Rufen	ANALGESIC	See *ibuprofen*.
salicylate	NSAI	See listing for **salicylsalicylic acid**.

salicylsalicylic acid
salsalate
   Disalcid
      NSAI, ANALGESIC, ANTIPYRETIC
      Drug: Take c̄ 8oz H_2O or milk. If GI distress, take c̄ food or milk. Swallow tab whole. **Diet:** May ↑ Vit K requirements. **GI:** N&v, GI distress, heartburn.[13] **S/Cond:** Limit caffeine: see Table p. 231. Limit alcohol. Caution c̄ diabetic: large doses may ↑ hypoglycemic effects. **Metab/Phys:** Na & H_2O retention.[13] No effects on platelet aggregation.
      Blood/Serum: ↓ T_4, ↑ or ↓ uric acid, ↓ K

Salutensin   ANTIHYPERTENSIVE c̄ DIURETIC
      See listing for *rauwolfia serpentina*.
      See listing for *hydrochlorothiazide*.

Sandimmune	IMMUNOSUPPRESSANT	See *cyclosporine*.
Sanorex	APPETITE SUPPRESSANT	See *mazindol*.
Sansert	ANTIMIGRAINE	See *methysergide maleate*.

scopolamine
   Transderm-Scop
      ANTIEMETIC, ANTIVERTIGO
      S/Cond: Caution c̄ lactation. Avoid alcohol. **Other:** <u>Drowsiness</u>, <u>dry mouth</u>, confusion, blurred vision, dizziness.

MEDICATION	CLASSIFICATION & DIETARY/RELATED SIGNIFICANCES

secobarbital
Seconal
Less than
5mg Na/dose

SEDATIVE
> **Drug:** Swallow tab whole. **Diet:** Supplements: Pyr — May ↓ drug effects.[14] **GI:** N&v. **S/Cond:** Caution c̄ lactation. Avoid alcohol. **Other:** Dizziness, drowsiness.
> **Blood/Serum:** ↓ bilirubin.

secobarbital sodium
Seconal sodium

SEDATIVE
> 9 mg Na/100 mg capsule.

Sectral

ANTIHYPERTENSIVE   See **acebutolol.**

Semilente insulin

ANTIDIABETIC   See **insulin.**

senna
Senokot
Suspension: 3.16gm
sucrose/5ml
Granules: 1.98gm
sucrose/3gm

LAXATIVE, STOOL SOFTENER
> **Drug:** Take at bedtime c̄ 8oz H_2O. Liquid: Take c̄ fruit juice or milk to mask taste. **Diet:** Encourage ↑ fluids unless otherwise directed. **Nutr:** Depletes fat, K & Ca. **GI:** N&v, GI pain.
> **Blood/Serum:** ↑ glucose, ↓ K (in extended use).

Septra

ANTIBIOTIC   See **trimethoprim c̄ sulfamethoxazole.**

Ser-Ap-Es *reserpine,* *hydralazine HCl,* *hydrochlorothiazide*	ANTIHYPERTENSIVE c̄ DIURETIC **Drug:** Take c̄ meals or milk to ↑ absorption & ↓ GI irritation. **Diet Important:** Possible ↓ Na, ↓ cal diet. May ↑ need for Pyr.[13] Avoid natural licorice. **GI:** ↑ GI motility; ↑ acid secretion. N&v, diarrhea. **S/Cond:** Not c̄ lactation. Avoid alcohol. Monitor diabetic: may alter insulin requirements. **Metab/Phys:** Monitor electrolytes. Anemias, edema. **Other:** <u>Drowsiness</u>, ↑ wt, dizziness, dry mouth, anorexia. **Blood/Serum:** ↑ glucose, ↑ uric acid, ↑ Ca, ↓ Na, ↓ K, ↓ Cl, ↓ Ⓟ, ↓ Mg. **Urinary:** ↑ Na, ↑ K, ↑ Cl, ↓ uric acid, ↓ Ca, ↑ bicarbonate, ↑ glucose, ↑ Mg.[3]	
Serax	ANTIANXIETY, benzodiazepine	15mg tab: tartrazine.[10] See ***oxazepam***.
Serentil	ANTIPSYCHOTIC	See ***mesoridazine***.
Seromycin	ANTIBIOTIC	See ***cycloserine***.
Serpasil	ANTIHYPERTENSIVE	See listing for ***rauwolfia serpentina***.

See "Guide to the Use of This Book" p. 5 for explanation of format.

MEDICATION	CLASSIFICATION & DIETARY/RELATED SIGNIFICANCES

simethicone
Mylicon

ANTIFLATULENT

> **Drug:** Take after meals or at bedtime. **Diet:** Proper diet & exercise important.[13] Avoid carbonated beverages & gas forming foods.

Sinemet

ANTIPARKINSONISM   See **levodopa & carbidopa.**

Sinequan

ANTIDEPRESSANT   See **doxepin HCl.**

Slo-phyllin 80
theophylline

ANTIASTHMA, BRONCHODILATOR   Suspension: 2.88gm sorbitol/5ml.
See **theophylline.**

Slow-K

ELECTROLYTE   See **potassium chloride.**

sodium bicarbonate
Sodium Bicarbonate
144mg Na/520mg tab
23mg Na/vial

ANTACID

> **Drug:** Take 1–3 hr after meals. **Diet:** Fe supplement: Concurrent intake ↓ Fe absorption; space doses.[13] **GI:** Belching, flatulence, gastric secretion & distention. **S/Cond:** Chronic use c̄ milk or Ca carbonate: ↑ Ca absorption & may precipitate milk-alkali syndrome.[13] Not c̄ ↓ Na diet. **Metab/Phys:** Edema. **Other:** ↑ wt.

Solu-Cortef
hydrocortisone
sodium succinate

CORTICOSTEROID   See **hydrocortisone.**

> **Drug:** Parenterally administered. 47.5mg Na/gm.
> **Diet:** May need ↓ Na, ↑ K diet.

Solu-Medrol *methylprednisolone sodium succinate*	CORTICOSTEROID **Drug:** Parenterally administered. 46.2mg Na/gm. **Diet:** May need ↓ Na, ↑ K diet.	See ***hydrocortisone.***
Soma	MUSCLE RELAXANT	See ***carisoprodol.***
Soma Compound c̄ codeine: 200mg carisoprodol 325mg aspirin 16mg codeine phosphate Contains sulfites	MUSCLE RELAXANT **Drug:** Take c̄ food if GI upset. **GI:** N&v, epigastric distress, constipation.[7] **S/Cond:** Not c̄ lactation. Avoid alcohol. **Other:** <u>Drowsiness</u>, dizziness, tremors, visual problems. **Blood/Serum:** ↑ amylase, ↑ lipase, ↑ or ↓ uric acid, ↓ T_4. **Urinary:** ↑ glucose (c̄ $CuSO_4$).[13]	
Somophylline	BRONCHODILATOR	See ***aminophylline.***
Sorbitrate	ANTIANGINAL	See ***isosorbide dinitrate.***
Spectrobid	ANTIBIOTIC, penicillin Suspension: 2.3 gm sucrose/5ml.	See ***bacampicillin.***

MEDICATION	CLASSIFICATION & DIETARY/RELATED SIGNIFICANCES

spironolactone
Aldactone

DIURETIC, POTASSIUM-SPARING PREPARATIONS
    Drug: Take c̄ food 6 or more hr before bedtime. **Diet Important:** Monitor K. Avoid natural licorice & salt substitutes.
    GI: Diarrhea, GI cramps. **S/Cond:** Not c̄ lactation. Caution c̄ diabetic: may ↑ serum glucose. **Metab/Phys:** Possible fluid & electrolyte imbalance. **Other:** Confusion, dry mouth, drowsiness, thirst, anorexia, altered taste.[37]
    Blood/Serum: ↑ K, ↑ BUN, ↓ Na, ↓ Cl, ↑ creatinine, ↑ Mg, ↑ uric acid.
    Urinary: ↑ Na, ↑ Cl, ↓ K, ↑ Mg, ↑ Ca.

spironolactone c̄
hydrochlorothiazide
Aldactazide

ANTIHYPERTENSIVE c̄ DIURETIC
    Drug: Take c̄ food 6 or more hr before bedtime. **Diet Important:** ↓ Na, ↓ cal diet may be recommended. Avoid natural licorice & salt substitutes. **GI:** GI cramps, diarrhea, n&v. **S/Cond:** Not c̄ lactation. Monitor diabetic: may alter serum glucose. Loss of appetite. **Metab/Phys:** Electrolyte imbalance. **Other:** Dry mouth, confusion, thirst, drowsiness.
    Blood/Serum: ↑ uric acid, ↑ Ca, ↑ BUN, ↑ K, ↑ or ↓ glucose, ↓ Na, ↓ Cl, ↓ bicarbonate, ↓ ℗, ↓ Zn.
    Urinary: ↑ Na, ↑ Cl, ↑ bicarbonate, ↑ uric acid, ↓ K, ↓ Ca, ↓ Thi, ↓ Pyr, ↓ ℗, ↓ Mg, ↑ Zn, ↑ Rib.

Staphcillin	ANTIBIOTIC, penicillin 67mg Na/1gm vial.	See ***methicillin sodium.***
Stelazine	ANTIPSYCHOTIC	See ***trifluoperazine HCl.***

streptozocin **Zanosar**
ANTINEOPLASTIC
Drug: Parenterally administered. **Diet:** Encourage ↑ fluids unless otherwise directed. **GI:** N&v, diarrhea. **S/Cond:** Monitor diabetic: ↓ CHO tolerance. **Other:** Confusion.
Blood/Serum: ↑ SGOT, ↑ LDH, ↓ albumin, ↑ BUN, ↑ bilirubin, ↑ SGPT, ↑ alk phos, ↓ Ⓟ, ↑ creatinine, ↓ glucose.[13]
Urinary: + protein.

sucralfate **Carafate**
ANTIULCER
Drug: Take tab c̄ H$_2$O on an empty stomach 1 hr before meals & at bedtime. **Nutr:** Interferes c̄ absorption of Vit A, D, E, & K. Long term use may cause deficiencies. **GI:** Constipation, diarrhea, GI cramps, nausea. **S/Cond:** Not c̄ lactation. **Other:** Dry mouth.

Sudafed	DECONGESTANT	See ***pseudoephedrine HCl.***

MEDICATION	CLASSIFICATION & DIETARY/RELATED SIGNIFICANCES

sulfamethoxazole
Gantanol
Suspension: 2.5gm
sucrose/5ml

ANTIBIOTIC, sulfonamide
Drug: Take c̄ 8oz H_2O on empty stomach.[13] **Diet:** Ensure adequate fluids. Supplements: PABA concurrent use ↓ activity of drug.[1]
Nutr: Interferes c̄ absorption of Fol, Vit B_{12}, K, Mg: advise good food sources. **GI:** N&v, stomatitis, diarrhea. **S/Cond:** Limit alcohol. Not c̄ lactation. **Metab/Phys:** Blood dyscrasias, pancreatitis.
Other: ↓ appetite, fatigue, dizziness.
Blood/Serum: ↑ creatinine.[3]
Urinary: ↑ Vit C,[11] ↑ glucose (false + c̄ $CuSO_4$).

sulfasalazine
Azulfidine
Contains sucrose

ANTIBIOTIC, sulfonamide
Drug: Take c̄ 8oz H_2O after meals. Do not crush. **Diet:** Encourage ↑ fluids unless otherwise directed. Need foods ↑ in Fol & Fe.
Nutr: ↓ absorption of Fe & Fol.[3] **GI:** N&v, abdominal pain, stomatitis, diarrhea. **S/Cond:** Caution c̄ diabetic. Caution c̄ lactation.
Metab/Phys: Blood dyscrasias, pancreatitis. **Other:** Anorexia, drowsiness, altered taste.[39]
Urinary: + for protein.

sulfinpyrazone
Anturane

ANTIGOUT, uricosuric, ANTIPLATELET
Drug: Take c̄ food or milk. **Diet:** ↑ fluid intake to 2.5–3qts/day in gout. More soluble in alkaline urine.[1] **GI:** GI distress, nausea.

S/Cond: Avoid alcohol. Monitor diabetic: ↑ insulin action. Not c̄ lactation. **Metab/Phys:** Blood dyscrasias. **Other:** Anorexia, sore throat.

sulfisoxazole **Gantrisin**	ANTIBIOTIC, sulfonamide	Syrup: 3.5gm sucrose/5ml. See listing for ***sulfamethoxazole.***

sulindac
Clinoril
ANTIARTHRITIC, NSAI
  Drug: Optimal: Take c̄ 8oz H$_2$O on empty stomach. May take c̄ food if GI upset. **GI:** Abdominal pain,[4] dyspepsia, flatulence, constipation, gastritis, n&v, diarrhea. **S/Cond:** Avoid alcohol. Not c̄ lactation. **Other:** Drowsiness, dizziness, headache.
  Blood/Serum: ↑ alk phos, ↑ SGOT, ↑ SGPT, ↑ K.
  Urinary: + protein.

Sumycin	ANTIBIOTIC	Syrup contains 2.2mg sucrose/5ml; sulfites. See ***tetracycline HCl.***
Surfak	STOOL SOFTENER	See ***docusate Ca.***
Symmetrel	ANTIPARKINSONISM, ANTIVIRAL	Syrup: 3.2 sorbitol/5ml. See ***amantadine HCl.***

MEDICATION	CLASSIFICATION & DIETARY/RELATED SIGNIFICANCES

Synalgos DC
dihydrocodeine
aspirin, caffeine
30mg caffeine/cap

ANALGESIC
   Drug: Take $\bar{c}$ food or 8oz H_2O. **GI:** N&v, constipation.
   S/Cond: Avoid alcohol. **Other:** Dizziness, drowsiness, dry mouth.
   Blood/Serum: ↑ or ↓ uric acid, dose-related, ↓ T_4, ↑ amylase,
   ↑ lipase.
   Urinary: ↑ glucose (false + $\bar{c}$ $CuSO_4$), ↓ bilirubin.

Synthroid
levothyroxine sodium

THYROID PREPARATION   Tartrazine: 0.1mg & 0.3mg tab.
                                 See listing for *thyroid.*

Tagamet

ANTIULCER   See *cimetidine.*

Talwin NX

ANALGESIC   See *pentazocine HCl.*

Tambocor

ANTIARRHYTHMIC   See *flecainide acetate.*

tamoxifen citrate
   Nolvadex

ANTINEOPLASTIC
   GI: N&v. **S/Cond:** Not $\bar{c}$ lactation. **Metab/Phys:** Edema, anemia,
   hypercalcemia.[7] **Other:** ↑ wt, altered taste, dizziness, blurred
   vision, ↓ appetite.[7]
   Blood/Serum: ↑ Ca.[3]

TAO

ANTIBIOTIC   See *troleandomycin.*

Tapazole	ANTITHYROID	See *methimazole*.
Tazidime	ANTIBIOTIC	See *ceftazidime*.

Tedral
theophylline
ephedrine HCl
phenobarbital
Elixir: 15% alcohol[10]

BRONCHODILATOR
    Drug: Take c̄ 8oz H_2O on empty stomach. Swallow tab whole.
    Diet: Limit charcoal broiled foods. **GI:** Epigastric distress.
    S/Cond: Limit alcohol. Limit caffeine: see Table p. 231.
    Other: Drowsiness, tremors.
    Blood/Serum: ↑ glucose.
    Urinary: albumin.

Teebacin	ANTITUBERCULAR	See *aminosalicylate Na*.
Tegopen	ANTIBIOTIC	14 mg NA/250 mg tablet. See *cloxacillin Na*.
Tegretol	ANTICONVULSANT	See *carbamazepine*.
Teldrin	ANTIHISTAMINIC	See *chlorpheniramine*.

temazepam
  Restoril

HYPNOTIC, benzodiazepine
    Drug: Swallow caps whole. **GI:** Diarrhea. **S/Cond:** Caution c̄ lactation. Avoid alcohol. **Other:** Drowsiness, dizziness, anorexia, confusion, tremors.

MEDICATION	CLASSIFICATION & DIETARY/RELATED SIGNIFICANCES

Tenex
ANTIHYPERTENSIVE See *guanfacine.*

Tenoretic
atenolol &
chlorthalidone
ANTIHYPERTENSIVF See *atenolol* & *chlorthalidone.*

Tenormin
ANTIHYPERTENSIVE See *atenolol.*

Tenuate
APPETITE SUPPRESSANT See *diethylpropion HCl.*

Tepanil
APPETITE SUPPRESSANT See *diethylpropion HCl.*

terazosin HCl
Hytrin
ANTIHYPERTENSIVE
> **Drug:** Take s̄ regard to food at the same time each day. **Diet Important:** ↓ Na, ↓ cal diet may be recommended. **GI:** Nausea. **S/Cond:** Caution c̄ lactation. **Metab/Phys:** Edema. **Other:** Dizziness, headache, blurred vision, sore throat.

terbutaline sulfate
Brethine
Bricanyl
ANTIASTHMA, BRONCHODILATOR
> **GI:** N&v. **S/Cond:** Caution c̄ diabetic. **Other:** Tremors, dizziness, headache, drowsiness.

tetracycline HCl
Achromycin-V
Cyclopar
ANTIBIOTIC
> **Drug:** Take c̄ 8oz H_2O on empty stomach. **Diet:** Do not give c̄ milk formulas or dairy products or Fe supplement within 2 hr. ↑ need

Sumycin
Tetracycline
Tetracyn

for Rib & Vit C.[15] Supplements: Vit A-Combination therapy may enhance drug-induced intracranial hypertension. Ca, Fe, Mg, or Zn-Concomitant intake may result in formation of insoluble complexes & impair both drug & Ca, Fe, Mg, or Zn absorption.[14]
Nutr: ↓ absorption of Ca, Fe, Zn & amino acids.[11] May ↓ absorption of fat & these nutrients may ↓ drug absorption.
GI: Diarrhea, n&v. **Metab/Phys:** ↓ bacterial synthesis of Vit K in intestines. **Other:** Anorexia, glossitis, altered taste.[37]
Blood/Serum: ↑ alk phos, ↑ BUN, ↑ amylase, ↑ bilirubin, ↑ SGOT, ↑ SGPT.

theophylline
Bronkodyl
Elixophyllin
Slophyllin-80
Theobid
Theodur
Theolair
Theo-24
Uniphyll

BRONCHODILATOR
Drug: For a uniform response, take sustained-release formulations consistently in relation to meals: a ↑ fat breakfast ↑ absorption c̄ some preparations & not others. Swallow cap/tab whole; chew chewables. **Diet:** Avoid extemes of dietary protein & CHO.[14] Limit charcoal broiled foods. **GI:** N&v, epigastric distress, diarrhea, hematemesis. **S/Cond:** Limit intake of caffeine-containing foods & beverages:[13] see Table p. 231. Caution c̄ lactation.
Metab/Phys: Inappropriate ADH syndrome.[10] Hyperglycemia.
Other: Dizziness, bitter aftertaste, headache.
Blood/Serum: ↑ glucose, ↑ uric acid, ↑ bilirubin.
Urinary: albumin.

MEDICATION	CLASSIFICATION & DIETARY/RELATED SIGNIFICANCES
theophylline & *guaifenesin*	BRONCHODILATOR, EXPECTORANT See listing for *theophylline.* See listing for *guaifenesin.*

thioridazine HCl
Mellaril
Concentrate: alcohol
Suspension: 3.16gm
   sucrose/5ml
	ANTIPSYCHOTIC
	    Drug: Take c̄ food. Swallow tab whole. **Diet:** ↑ need for Rib.
	    GI: Constipation, n&v, diarrhea. **S/Cond:** Avoid alcohol.
	    Metab/Phys: Edema, anemia. **Other:** <u>Dry mouth</u>, <u>drowsiness</u>,
	    <u>↑ wt</u>, blurred vision, dizziness.
	    <u>**Urinary:** ↑</u> bilirubin (false elevation).

thiothixene
Navane
	ANTIPSYCHOTIC
	    Drug: Take c̄ food or H_2O. **GI:** N&v, constipation, diarrhea.
	    S/Cond: Limit alcohol. **Metab/Phys:** Blood dyscrasias, edema.
	    Other: Drowsiness, dizziness, dry mouth, blurred vision, ↑ wt,
	    ↑ appetite, tremors, ↑ salivation.
	    Blood/Serum: ↑ alk phos, ↑ SGOT, ↑ SGPT, ↓ uric acid.

Thorazine	ANTIPSYCHOTIC See *chlorpromazine HCl.*

thyroglobulin
  Proloid
thyroid
  Thyroid

THYROID PREPARATION
  Drug: Take on empty stomach to ↑ absorption.[1] **Diet:** Limit intake of foods containing goitrogens: see Table p. 236. Ineffective for wt loss. **GI:** N&v, diarrhea, epigastric distress. **S/Cond:** Monitor diabetic: possible ↓ glucose tolerance. **Other:** ↓ wt, headache.
  Blood/Serum: ↑ glucose, ↑ T_4.
  Urinary: + glucose.[3]

Thyrolar
  liotrix

THYROID PREPARATION   See listing for ***thyroid***.

ticarcillin disodium
  Ticar
  Powder:
    120-150mg Na/gm

ANTIBIOTIC, penicillin
  Drug: Parenterally administered. **GI:** N&v. **S/Cond:** Caution c̄ lactation. **Metab/Phys:** Monitor electrolytes: ↑ Na, ↓ K.
  Blood/Serum: ↑ SGOT, ↑ SGPT.

Tigan

ANTINAUSEANT, ANTIEMETIC   See ***trimethobenzamide HCl***.

Timentin
  ticarcillin disodium & clavulante K
  10 9mg Na/gm,
  6mg K/100mg

ANTIBIOTIC, penicillin
  Diet: Parenterally administered. **GI:** N&v, flatulence, diarrhea, epigastric pain, stomatitis. **S/Cond:** Caution c̄ lactation.
  Metab/Phys: Monitor electrolytes: ↑ Na, ↓ K, anemia.
  Other: Headache, altered taste & smell.
  Blood/Serum: ↑ SGOT, ↑ SGPT, ↑ alk phos, ↑ LDH, ↑ bilirubin, ↑ creatinine, ↑ BUN, ↑ Na, ↓ K, ↓ uric acid.

MEDICATION	CLASSIFICATION & DIETARY/RELATED SIGNIFICANCES

timolol maleate
Blocadren

ANTIHYPERTENSIVE, beta blocker
    Drug: Take c̄ food same time each day. **Diet Important:** ↓ Na,
↓ cal may be recommended. Avoid natural licorice. **GI:** Nausea.
S/Cond: Not c̄ lactation. Caution diabetic: may mask signs of
hypoglycemia.[1] **Metab/Phys:** Edema. **Other:** Fatigue, dizziness, visual problems, ↓ wt, headache.
Blood/Serum: ↑ BUN, ↑ K, ↑ uric acid, ↑ or ↓ glucose,
↑ TG, ↓ HDL.

tobramycin sulfate
Nebcin

ANTIBIOTIC, aminoglycoside
    Drug: Parenterally administered. **Diet:** Encourage ↑ fluids
unless otherwise directed. **GI:** N&v. **Metab/Phys:** Anemia.
Other: Anorexia, dizziness, headache, confusion.
Blood/Serum: ↑ BUN, ↑ SGOT, ↑ SGPT, ↑ LDH, ↑ bilirubin,
↑ creatinine, ↓ Mg, ↓ Na, ↓ K, ↓ Ca.
Urinary: ↑ Mg, ↑ K, + protein.

tocainide HCl
Tonocard

ANTIARRHYTHMIC
    Drug: Take c̄ food. **GI:** N&v, diarrhea. **S/Cond:** Not c̄ lactation.
Metab/Phys: Blood dyscrasias. **Other:** Dizziness, tremors, headache, drowsiness, ↓ appetite, dry mouth.

Tofranil	ANTIDEPRESSANT	See *imipramine HCl.*

tolazamide
Tolinase   ORAL HYPOGLYCEMIC   See listing for *tolbutamide.*

tolbutamide
Orinase   ORAL HYPOGLYCEMIC
  Drug: Take in AM or divided during day c̄ prescribed diet plan.
  Diet: Compliance Important. Not a substitute for dietary regulation.
  GI: Diarrhea, GI distress, n&v, dyspepsia, heartburn. **S/Cond:** Avoid alcohol: possible disulfiram-like reaction.[7] **Other:** Altered taste, ↓ appetite, headache.
  Blood/Serum: ↓ glucose.
  Urinary: ↓ glucose.

tolmetin sodium
Tolectin
36mg Na/tab   NSAI, ANTIARTHRITIC
  Drug: May take c̄ meals. **GI:** N&v, dyspepsia, GI distress, diarrhea, constipation, flatulence, gastric bleeding, gastritis. **S/Cond:** Not c̄ lactation. **Metab/Phys:** Edema. **Other:** Dizziness, drowsiness.
  Blood/Serum: ↑ Na, ↑ SGPT, ↑ SGOT, ↑ BUN.
  Urinary: + protein.

Totacillin   ANTIBIOTIC, penicillin   See *ampicillin.*
  Suspension: 1.8gm sucrose/5ml; 62–78mg Na/gm.

MEDICATION	CLASSIFICATION & DIETARY/RELATED SIGNIFICANCES

Trandate   ANTIHYPERTENSIVE   See *labetalol HCl.*

Transderm-Nitro   ANTIANGINAL   See *nitroglycerin.*

Transderm-Scop   ANTIEMETIC   See *scopolamine.*

Tranxene   ANTIANXIETY   See *clorazepate dipotassium.*

tranylcypromine sulfate
Parnate

ANTIDEPRESSANT, MAOI
Diet Important: Avoid foods ↑ in pressor agents;[3] see Table p. 234. Supplements: tryptophan — concurrent administration may result in hyperexcitability, headache, hypertension & hallucinations.[14] **GI:** Constipation, GI distress. **S/Cond:** Limit caffeine-containing foods & beverages: see Table p. 231. Avoid alcohol. Monitor diabetic: may alter glucose tolerance. **Metab/Phys:** Possible fluid & electrolyte imbalance. Edema. **Other:** Dizziness, drowsiness, ↓ or ↑ wt, tremors, dry mouth, blurred vision. **Blood/Serum:** ↓ glucose.

trazodone HCl
Desyrel
Trialodone
50mg tab: lactose

ANTIDEPRESSANT
Drug: Take c̄ food. **GI:** Flatulence. **S/Cond:** Not c̄ lactation. Limit alcohol. **Metab/Phys:** Anemia. **Other:** ↑ or ↓ appetite, altered taste, ↑ salivation, headache,[10] blurred vision, dry mouth.

Trental	HEMORRHEOLOGIC	See *pentoxifylline.*
Trexan	NARCOTIC DETERRENT	See *naltrexone.*

triamcinolone
  Aristocort
  Kenalog-40

CORTICOSTEROID   See listing for *hydrocortisone.*
    Drug: Parenterally or orally administered. **S/Cond:** Latent diabetes may be activated. **Other:** ↓ appetite ↓ wt.

Triaminic
  phenylpropanolamine HCl, pheniramine maleate, pyrilamine
  Expectorant:
    5% alcohol

ANTIHISTAMINIC, DECONGESTANT
    Drug: May take c̄ food, milk or H_2O. Swallow time-released cap whole. **GI:** Epigastric distress, n&v. **S/Cond:** Not c̄ lactation. Avoid alcohol. Caution c̄ diabetic. **Other:** Blurred vision, dizziness, drowsiness, sedation, possible unusual excitement (especially in children),[13] disturbed coordination, dry mouth, altered taste.

triamterene
  Dyrenium

DIURETIC
    Drug: Take c̄ food. **Diet:** Avoid salt substitutes & diets ↑ in K. Supplements: Fol — ↓ utilization of dietary Fol.[9] **Nutr:** May ↓ serum Fol, ↑ Ca excretion. Conserves K. **GI:** N&v, diarrhea, GI distress. **S/Cond:** Not c̄ lactation. Monitor diabetic: possible ↑ blood glucose level. **Metab/Phys:** Blood dyscrasias. **Other:** Dry mouth, headache.
    Blood/Serum: ↑ uric acid, ↑ LDH, ↓ Na, ↑ K, ↓ Cl.
    Urinary: ↑ Na, ↓ K, ↑ Cl, ↑ uric acid.

See "Guide to the Use of This Book" p. 5 for explanation of format.

MEDICATION	CLASSIFICATION & DIETARY/RELATED SIGNIFICANCES

triamterene c̄
hydrochlorothiazide
Dyazide
Maxzide

ANTIHYPERTENSIVE, DIURETIC
    Drug: Take c̄ food or milk 6 or more hr before bedtime. **Diet Important:** ↓ Na, ↓ cal diet may be needed. If on ↓ Na diet, monitor Na. **GI:** N&v, diarrhea, constipation. **S/Cond:** Not c̄ lactation. Limit alcohol. Monitor diabetic: may alter blood glucose levels. **Metab/Phys:** Electrolyte imbalance, monitor K. Blood dyscrasias, pancreatitis, jaundice. **Other:** Dry mouth, thirst, dehydration.
    Blood/Serum: ↓ Fol, ↑ uric acid, ↑ Ca, ↓ Na, ↑ K, ↓ Cl, ↑ creatinine, ↑ BUN, ↑ or ↓ glucose.
    Urinary: ↑ Na, ↓ K, ↑ Cl, ↑ uric acid, ↑ bicarbonate, ↓ Ca, ↑ Fol, ↑ glucose.

Triavil

ANTIDEPRESSANT   See *perphenazine.*
                                   See *amitriptyline HCl.*

triazolam
Halcion

SEDATIVE, benzodiazepine
    Drug: Take at bedtime. **GI:** N&v, constipation. **S/Cond:** Not c̄ lactation. Avoid alcohol. **Other:** Drowsiness, dizziness, headache, altered taste, dry mouth, confusion.

Tribavirin

ANTIVIRAL   See *ribavirin.*

trifluoperazine HCl
Stelazine
Liquid contains sulfites

ANTIPSYCHOTIC
Drug: Take c̄ food to ↓ GI irritation. To take concentrate, add to liquid or foods. **Diet:** ↑ need of Rib.[13] **Nutr:** May ↓ absorption of Vit B_{12}.[16] **GI:** Constipation. **S/Cond:** Not c̄ lactation. Avoid alcohol. **Metab/Phys:** Edema, blood dyscrasias. **Other:** Drowsiness, dizziness, dry mouth, blurred vision, ↑ appetite, ↑ wt.
Blood/Serum: ↑ SGOT, ↑ SGPT, ↑ LDH, ↑ alk phos, ↑ bilirubin, ↑ or ↓ glucose.
Urinary: + glucose, + bilirubin.

triflupromazine HCl
Vesprin
25mg & 50mg tab: tartrazine[3]

ANTIPSYCHOTIC, ANTINAUSEANT
Drug: Take c̄ food, milk or 8oz H_2O. **Diet:** May ↑ need for Rib.[13] **Nutr:** May ↓ absorption of B_{12}.[16] **GI:** Constipation. **S/Cond:** Limit alcohol. **Metab/Phys:** Blood dyscrasias, peripheral edema, jaundice. **Other:** Drowsiness, dry mouth, dizziness, lethargy, anorexia, ↑ or ↓ wt, tremors.
Blood/Serum: ↑ SGOT, ↑ SGPT, ↑ LDH, ↑ alk phos, ↓ bilirubin.
Urinary: + bilirubin.

MEDICATION	CLASSIFICATION & DIETARY/RELATED SIGNIFICANCES

trihexyphenidyl HCl
Artane
Elixir: sucrose,
5% alcohol

ANTIPARKINSONISM
Drug: Take c̄ food to ↓ GI irritation. Swallow sustained release cap whole. Do not crush. **GI:** N&v, constipation. **S/Cond:** Avoid alcohol. **Other:** Dry mouth, blurred vision, anorexia, drowsiness, weakness.

Trilafon

ANTIPSYCHOTIC   See *perphenazine.*

trimethobenzamide HCl
Tigan
Contains lactose

ANTINAUSEANT, ANTIEMETIC
GI: Diarrhea. **S/Cond:** Avoid alcohol. **Metab/Phys:** Blood dyscrasias, jaundice.[10] **Other:** Drowsiness, tremors, dizziness, sore throat, blurred vision, headache.

trimethoprim c̄
sulfamethoxazole
Bactrim
Suspension: 2.5mg
sucrose/5ml

Septra
Suspension: 3.5gm
sucrose/5ml

ANTIBIOTIC, sulfonamide
Drug: Take c̄ 8oz H_2O on empty stomach. **Diet:** Encourage ↑ fluids unless otherwise directed. **Nutr:** ↓ absorption of Fol.[11] ↓ absorption of Vit K in long term use.[12] **GI:** Diarrhea, stomatitis, GI distress. **S/Cond:** Not c̄ lactation. Caution diabetic: rare hypoglycemia.[13] **Metab/Phys:** Caution c̄ G6PD. Anemias, jaundice, hepatitis. **Other:** Dizziness, anorexia.
Blood/Serum: ↑ creatinine, ↑ BUN, ↑ SGOT, ↑ SGPT, ↑ bilirubin.
Urinary: ↑ Vit C.[11]

Trimox	ANTIBIOTIC	See *amoxicillin*.

Trinalin
azatadine maleate, pseudoephedrine sulfate

ANTIHISTAMINIC, DECONGESTANT
Drug: May take c̄ food, H_2O or milk. Swallow tab whole.
GI: Epigastric distress, n&v, diarrhea, constipation. **S/Cond:** Not c̄ lactation. Caution c̄ diabetics: may alter blood glucose levels. Avoid alcohol. **Metab/Phys:** Anemias. **Other:** Sedation, disturbed coordination, dry mouth, confusion, anorexia, blurred vision.

Trinsicon
Vit B_{12}, ferrous fumarate, Vit C, Fol & intrinsic factor

HEMATINIC
Drug: Optimal: Take c̄ 8oz H_2O on empty stomach: food ↓ absorption. **GI:** GI distress, diarrhea, constipation, nausea, heartburn. **S/Cond:** Caution c̄ lactation.

troleandomycin
  TAO
  Cap: lactose[10]

ANTIBIOTIC
Drug: Take 1 hr before or 2 hr after meals. **Diet:** Acid stable.
GI: Abdominal cramps, n&v, diarrhea. **S/Cond:** Caution c̄ lactation.
Metab/Phys: Jaundice.

Tums	ANTACID	See *calcium carbonate*.
Tylenol	ANALGESIC	See *acetaminophen*.

See "Guide to the Use of This Book" p. 5 for explanation of format.

MEDICATION	CLASSIFICATION & DIETARY/RELATED SIGNIFICANCES	
Tylenol c̄ Codeine *codeine phosphate,* *acetaminophen*	ANALGESIC, NARCOTIC Elixir: 7% alcohol; 3mg sucrose/5ml. See *acetaminophen.* See listing for *codeine.*	
Tylox *oxycodone HCl &* *acetaminophen*	ANALGESIC, NARCOTIC	See *Percocet.*
Ultracef	ANTIBIOTIC, cephalosporin	Suspension: 3gm sucrose/5ml. See *cefadroxil.*
Ultralente Insulin beef & pork, or beef	ANTIDIABETIC	See *insulin.*
Unipen	ANTIBIOTIC	See *nafcillin Na.*
Uniphyll	BRONCHODILATOR	See *theophylline.*
Urecholine	CHOLINERGIC	See *bethanechol chloride.*
Urex	ANTI-INFECTIVE	See *methenamine hippurate.*

Urised
atropine sulfate,
hyoscyamine,
methenamine,
methylene blue,
phenyl salicylate &
benzoic acid

ANTI-INFECTIVE, ANTISPASMODIC, urinary
 Drug: Take c̄ 8oz H_2O.[3] May take c̄ food to ↓ GI upset.
 Diet: Drink adequate fluids; do not over-hydrate. Drug most effective c̄ urine of 5.5 pH or ↓. Avoid excessive intake of alkalinizing foods:[7] see Table p. 238. **GI:** N&v, stomach pain, diarrhea.
 Other: Dry mouth, blurred vision, dizziness, drowsiness, ↓ appetite.[13]

Urispas	ANTISPASMODIC	See *flavoxate HCl.*
Utimox	ANTIBIOTIC	See *amoxicillin.*
Valium	ANTIANXIETY	See *diazepam.*
Valmid	HYPNOTIC	See *ethinamate.*

valproic acid
 Depakene

ANTICONVULSANT
 Drug: Take after meals to ↓ GI distress. Swallow cap whole. Do not take oral solution c̄ carbonated beverages. **GI:** N&v, indigestion, abdominal pain, constipation, diarrhea. **S/Cond:** Avoid alcohol. Caution c̄ lactation. **Metab/Phys:** ↓ plasma Ca, ↓ plasma P, bone changes. Anemia. **Other:** ↑ or ↓ appetite, ↑ or ↓ wt, tremors, sedation, headache, dizziness.
 Blood/Serum: ↑ alk phos, ↑ SGOT, ↑ SGPT, ↑ bilirubin, ↑ LDH (dose related), ↑ or ↓ uric acid (dose related), altered thyroid tests.
 Urinary: ± ketones.

MEDICATION	CLASSIFICATION & DIETARY/RELATED SIGNIFICANCES

vancomycin HCl
Vancocin
	ANTIBIOTIC
	    Drug: Parenterally or orally administered. **GI:** N&v.
	    S/Cond: Caution c̄ lactation. **Other:** Bitter taste, weakness, thirst,
	    ↓ appetite.

Vasotec	ANTIHYPERTENSIVE See *enalapril maleate.*
Vee-Tids	ANTIBIOTIC See *penicillin.*
Velban	ANTINEOPLASTIC See *vinblastine sulfate.*
Velosef	ANTIBIOTIC See *cephradine.*
Velosulin *insulin, pork*	ANTIDIABETIC See *insulin.*
Ventolin	BRONCHODILATOR See *albuterol sulfate.*

verapamil HCl
  Calan
  Isoptin
	ANTIARRHYTHMIC, Ca-channel blocker
	    Drug: Take sustained released tab c̄ food or milk. Other formula-
	    tions: Take s̄ regard to meals.[3] **GI:** Constipation. **S/Cond:** Not c̄ lac-
	    tation. Avoid alcohol. Caution c̄ diabetic.[9] **Metab/Phys:** Edema.
	    Other: Dizziness, headache, fatigue.
	    Blood/Serum: ↑ SGOT, ↑ SGPT, ↑ alk phos, ↑ bilirubin.[3]

VePesid	ANTINEOPLASTIC	See *etoposide*.
Vesprin	ANTIPSYCHOTIC	See *triflupromazine HCl*.
Vibramycin	ANTIBIOTIC	See *doxycycline*.

Vicodin
hydrocodone bitartrate & acetaminophen
    ANALGESIC, NARCOTIC, ANTITUSSIVE
    GI: N&v, constipation. **S/Cond:** Not c̄ lactation. Avoid alcohol.
    Other: Drowsiness, dizziness, dry mouth.
    Blood/Serum: ↑ amylase, ↑ lipase, ↓ glucose.

vidarabine monohydrate
  Vira-A
    ANTIVIRAL
    Drug: Parenterally administered. **GI:** N&v, diarrhea. **S/Cond:** Not c̄ lactation. **Other:** Anorexia, tremors, confusion, ↓ wt, dizziness.
    Blood/Serum: ↑ SGOT, ↑ bilirubin, ↓ Hb, ↓ HCT.[7]

vinblastine sulfate
  Velban
    ANTINEOPLASTIC
    Drug: Parenterally administered. **Diet:** Encourage ↑ fluids unless otherwise directed. Need snacks of ↑ nutrient density.
    GI: N&v, abdominal pain, diarrhea, constipation, stomatitis.
    Metab/Phys: Leukopenia. **Other:** Anorexia, sore throat, weakness, dizziness, headache.
    Blood/Serum: ↑ uric acid.
    Urinary: ↑ uric acid.

214

MEDICATION	CLASSIFICATION & DIETARY/RELATED SIGNIFICANCES

vincristine sulfate
  Oncovin

ANTINEOPLASTIC
    Drug: Parenterally administered. **Diet:** Encourage ↑ fluids unless otherwise directed. **GI:** <u>Constipation</u>, stomach pain, n&v.
    Metab/Phys: ↑ release of ADH: possible hyponatremia. Anemia.
    Other: Thirst, mouth sores/ulcers, ↓ wt, double vision, muscle wasting, altered taste.[37]
    Blood/Serum: ↑ K, ↑ uric acid.
    Urinary: ↑ uric acid.

Vira-A	ANTIVIRAL	See *vidarabine monohydrate.*
Virazole	ANTIVIRAL	See *ribavirin.*
Visken	ANTIHYPERTENSIVE	See *pindolol.*
Vistaril	ANTIANXIETY	See *hydroxyzine HCl.*
Vivactil	ANTIDEPRESSANT	See *protriptyline HCl.*

warfarin sodium **Coumadin**	ANTICOAGULANT	

Diet: Parenterally or orally administered. **Diet:** Balanced diet $\bar{c}$ consistent intake of Vit K: ↑ K, ↓ drug effectiveness.[15] See Table p. 236. Limit green teas & herbal teas, see Table p. 232. Caution $\bar{c}$ fish oil supplements. Avoid proteolytic enzymes (papain), soybean oil,[8] fried or boiled onions, which ↑ fibrinolytic activity & ↑ drug action.[39] Large amounts of Vit A, E, K & C supplements alter prothrombin time. **Nutr:** Cooking oils $\bar{c}$ silicone additive ↓ drug absorption. **GI:** GI pain, n&v, constipation. **S/Cond:** Limit caffeine: see Table p. 231. Not $\bar{c}$ lactation. Avoid alcohol. **Other:** Bloating.

Wyamycin	ANTIBIOTIC	See ***erythromycin***.
Wymox	ANTIBIOTIC	See ***amoxicillin***.
Xanax	ANTIANXIETY	See ***alprazolam***.
Zanosar	ANTINEOPLASTIC	See ***streptozocin***.
Zantac	ANTIULCER	See ***ranitidine***.
Zarontin	ANTICONVULSANT	See ***ethosuximide***.
Zaroxolyn	DIURETIC	See ***metolazone***.

MEDICATION	CLASSIFICATION & DIETARY/RELATED SIGNIFICANCES	
Zestril	ANTIHYPERTENSIVE	See *lisinopril.*
zidovudine **AZT** **Retrovir**	ANTIVIRAL **GI:** Constipation, diarrhea. **Metab/Phys:** Anemias. **Other:** Altered taste, edema of tongue & lips, mouth ulcers, unusual tiredness, tremors, ↓ appetite.	
Zinacef	ANTIBIOTIC	54.2mg Na/gm. See *cefuroxime sodium.*
Zovirax	ANTIVIRAL	See *acyclovir.*
Zyloprim	ANTIGOUT	See *allopurinol.*

LABORATORY VALUES

These tests may alert the clinician to problems of nutritional significance. Value will depend on the analytical method employed and the procedure used by the individual laboratory. Results can be influenced by many factors and always must be interpreted by supportive clinical information. Values are for blood/serum unless otherwise stated.

CONSTITUENT	NORMAL VALUES (METHOD DEPENDENT)	SIGNIFICANCE OF ABNORMAL VALUES
Acetone, urine	0	↑ in impaired glucose metabolism; starvation
* Alkaline Phosphatase *alk phos*	1.5–4.5U/dl (Bodansky)	↑ liver disease, bone growth, osteomalacia, Hodgkin's disease, rickets, any tissue destruction, peptic ulcer, ulcerative colitis, hyperthyroidism, congestive heart failure, bone metastases, Paget's disease, pregnancy, cirrhosis, Ca deficiency, vitamin therapy ↓ in hypothyroidism, ↓ P diet, ↓ Vit C diet, cretinism, celiac disease, excessive Vit D therapy, scurvy, malnutrition, pernicious anemia

CONSTITUENT		NORMAL VALUES (METHOD DEPENDENT)	SIGNIFICANCE OF ABNORMAL VALUES
Albumin		3.0–5.5g/dl	↑ in dehydration, multiple myeloma, transfusions ↓ TB, cancer, stress, chronic infection, liver disease, burns, nephrotic syndrome, overhydration, eclampsia, protein-cal malnutrition, impaired digestion
Ammonia		80–110μg/dl	↑ liver disease
Amylase		53–123U/L	↑ acute pancreatitis, mumps; ↑ occasionally in renal insufficiency ↓ in hepatitis, pancreatic insufficiency
Ascorbic Acid		0.2–1.5mg/dl	↑ oxalate stones, diarrhea, ↑ uric acid ↓ causes delayed wound healing, scurvy, loose teeth, c̄ large doses of aspirin, oral contraceptives
Bilirubin	Direct Total	≤ 0.4mg/dl ≤ 1mg/dl	↑ chronic, acute, hepatitis, biliary obstruction, drug toxicity, jaundice, hemolytic disease, prolonged fasting

Blood Urea Nitrogen *BUN*	8–23mg/dl	↑ renal insufficiency-renal failure, myocardial failure, GI bleeding, fever, nephritis, malignancy, dehydration, excessive protein intake, shock ↓ hepatic failure, nephrosis, cachexia, overhydration, acute low protein intake, low protein-high CHO diet, malabsorption
Calcium	8.5–10.5mg/dl	↑ hyperparathyroidism, c̄ renal calculi, Vit D excess, osteolytic disease, milk-alkali syndrome, immobilization, TB, Addison's disease ↓ steatorrhea, severe nephritis, malabsorption syndrome, Vit D deficiency, hypoparathyroidism, sprue, celiac disease
Carbon Dioxide CO_2	24–30mEq/L	↑ pulmonary problems, in metabolic alkalosis due to ingestion of excess sodium bicarbonate, protracted vomiting c̄ K deficit, Cushing's syndrome, heart failure c̄ edema ↓ in diabetic ketosis, starvation, renal insufficiency, persistent diarrhea, lactic acidosis, respiratory alkalosis

CONSTITUENT	NORMAL VALUES (METHOD DEPENDENT)	SIGNIFICANCE OF ABNORMAL VALUES
Chloride	100–106mEq/L	↑ excessive salt intake, anxiety states, dehydration, fever, nephrosis, renal insufficiency, aspirin toxicity ↓ diabetic acidosis, metabolic alkalosis, vomiting, K deficiency, excessive sweating
* Cholesterol *chol*	150–250mg/dl	↑ in hyperlipemia, hypoproteinemia, pancreatitis, pancreatectomy, poorly controlled diabetes, liver disease c̄ biliary obstruction, hypothyroidism, glomerulonephritis ↓ acute infection, extensive liver disease, anemias, TB, starvation, cancer, malnutrition, certain enzyme deficiencies
* Copper *Cu*	70–150μg/dl	↑ in myocardial infarction, glomerulonephritis, malignant lymphoma, rheumatoid arthritis, cirrhosis of the liver, infections, pregnancy, anemias, hypo/hyper-thyroidism. Nonceruloplasmin Cu ↑ in Wilson's disease. Total serum Cu ↓ in Wilson's disease, nephrotic syndrome

Creatinine *creatine kinase* *(CK)*	0.7–1.5mg/dl	↑ muscle damage, myocardial infarction, muscular dystrophy, in acute & chronic renal insufficiency, urinary tract obstructions, & c̄ decreased glomerular filtration rate, fever, burns
GGT *gamma glutamyl* *transpeptidase*	0–65U/L	↑ liver disease ↑ hepatic biliary disease, pancreatitis, sensitive to post-op alcoholism
* Globulin	2.3–3.5g/dl	↑ in infections, liver disease, leukemia, hepatic disease, hyperlipidemia ↓ malnutrition
Glucose	70–110mg/dl	↑ in diabetes mellitus, chronic hepatic dysfunction, dehydration, hyperthyroidism, Vit B deficiency, diuretics, pancreatic insufficiency, acute stress, Cushing's syndrome, burns ↓ in hyperinsulinism, large, non-pancreatic tumors, pituitary dysfunction (exogenous or endogenous), carcinoma, pancreatic disorders, Addison's disease, ETOH abuse, extensive liver disease, functional hypoglycemia(?), malnutrition

CONSTITUENT	NORMAL VALUES (METHOD DEPENDENT)	SIGNIFICANCE OF ABNORMAL VALUES
* Hematocrit (HCT)	Female 37%–47% Male 45%–52%	↑ in polycythemia, dehydration, sickle-cell anemia, severe pancreatitis
* Hemoglobin (Hb)	Female 12–16g/dl Male 13–18g/dl	↓ in prolonged dietary deficiency of Fe ↓ in anemia c̄ GI blood loss
HDL Cholesterol *HDL*	30–80mg/dl	↑ vigorous exercise, estrogen or insulin therapy, some alcohol consumption ↓ starvation, obesity, liver disease, diabetes
* Iron *Fe*	40–160μg/dl	↑ excessive intake of Fe, hemolysis, liver disease, anemias ↓ Fe deficiency anemias, chronic infection, carcinoma, chronic liver disease, chronic renal insufficiency
Ketones, urine	0	↑ diabetic ketoacidosis, starvation, prolonged vomiting, toxemia, ↑ fat or ↓ carbohydrate diet, fever, thyrotoxicosis, Gierke's disease

Lactic Dehydrogenase *LDH (LD)*	45–90U/L	↑ cirrhosis, acute hepatitis, hemolytic disorders, pernicious anemia, myocardial infarction, progressive muscular dystrophy, burns, trauma, nephrotic syndrome
Lead, urine	≤ 50μg/dl	↑ in poisoning
Lipase	< 1.5 IU/ml	↑ in pancreatitis, biliary tract infection, renal insufficiency
Lipids, total	450–1000mg/dl	↑ in diabetes, biliary cirrhosis, nephrotic syndrome, xanthomatosis
Magnesium *Mg*	1.5–2mEq/L	↑ liver disease & overtreatment c̄ Mg salts ↓ ETOH abuse, starvation, prolonged IV therapy, drug therapy, diarrhea, vomiting, hepatic insufficiency
* Mean Corpuscular Volume (MCV)	86–98μm^3/cell	↑ ETOH abuse, macrocytic anemia of folic acid.

CONSTITUENT	NORMAL VALUES (METHOD DEPENDENT)	SIGNIFICANCE OF ABNORMAL VALUES
pH	7.35–7.45	↓ diabetic ketoacidosis, starvation, uremia, renal acidosis, ↑ protein or ↑ fat diet, acidic drugs ↑ metabolic alkalosis, hyperventilation, vomiting, alkali administration
Phosphate, inorganic Ⓟ	2.5–4.5mg/dl	↑ hypervitaminosis D, renal insufficiency, hypoparathyroidism, nephritis, Mg deficiency, bone disease ↓ hyperparathyroidism, osteomalacia, hyperinsulinism, antacid overuse, hypovitaminosis D, ideopathic steatorrhea, gout
Potassium K	3.5–5mEq/L	↑ in renal insufficiency, circulatory failure, tissue destruction, shock, Addison's disease, dehydration, ↓ diuretic therapy, ETOH abuse, vomiting, diarrhea, starvation, chronic stress, correction of diabetic acidosis, hypomagnesemia, Cushing's syndrome, malabsorption, laxative abuse
Protein, total	6–8.4g/dl	↑ in dehydration, malignancy, Hodgkin's disease, hepatitis, leukemia, acute or chronic infectious disease ↓ in malnutrition, malabsorption, cirrhosis, steatorrhea, edema, laxative use, marasmus, leukemia

* Red Blood Cells *erythrocytes* *RBC*	4.2–5.6mil/mm^3	↑ in polycythemia, dehydration ↓ anemia, hemorrhage, chronic infectious disease, prolonged dietary deficiency of Fe
SGOT (AST) *serum glutamic oxaloacetic transaminase*	7–27 U/L	↑ cirrhosis of liver, neoplastic disease, acute infections, acute hepatitis, burns, trauma, myocardial infarction ↓ Pyr deficiency, beriberi, chronic dialysis(?)
SGPT (ALT) *serum glutamic pyruvic transaminase*	1–21 U/L	↑ acute hepatitis, cirrhosis of liver, neoplastic disease
Sodium *Na*	135–145mEq/L	↑ dehydration, diabetes insipidus, steroid administration ↓ inappropriate anti-diuretic hormone (ADH), diuretic, burns, diarrhea, Addison's disease, chronic nephropathy, nephritis, starvation, diabetic acidosis, adrenal insufficiency, hyperlipidemia, hyperglycemia, hyperproteinemia ↓ in H$_2$O intoxication

CONSTITUENT	NORMAL VALUES (METHOD DEPENDENT)	SIGNIFICANCE OF ABNORMAL VALUES
Specific Gravity, urine	1.005–1.030	↑ fever, acute glomerulonephritis, nephrosis, toxemia, ↓ fluid intake, ↓ chronic glomerulonephritis or pyelonephritis, systemic lupus erythematosus, parenteral nutrition, ↑ fluid intake, hypothermia, diabetes insipidus
Thyroxine T_4 T_3	$4-12\mu g/100ml$ $75-195ng/100ml$	↑ hyperthyroidism, nephrosis, anticoagulant therapy ↓ estrogen therapy, hypothyroidism, nephrosis, cirrhosis
Triglycerides TG	40–150mg/dl	↑ liver diseases, gout, pancreatitis, ↑ ETOH abuse, hyperlipoproteinemia, myocardial infarction ↓ in malnutrition, malabsorption
Uric Acid	3.7mg/dl	↑ gout, renal insufficiency, lead poisoning, arthritis, high protein diets, starvation, leukemias, multiple myeloma, thiazide diuretics, hypoparathyroidism, ETOH abuse, anemia, psoriasis ↓ in high doses of salicylates, ↑ patients $\bar{c}$ arteriosclerosis, hypertension, and ↑ triglycerides

| * White Blood Cells
leukocytes
WBC | 4.5–10.6
thous/mm^3 | ↑ leukemias, acute infections, inflammations, fever, anemias
↓ chemotherapy |
| Zinc
Zn | 101–139μg/100ml | ↓ slow wound healing, hypogensia, growth restriction, alcoholic cirrhosis |

* These tests indicate a possible blood dyscrasia (any abnormal or pathological condition of the blood)

References: 32, 44, 7, 45

TESTS FOR MALABSORPTION

The following blood levels may be reduced below the usual norm in malabsorption disorders:
Blood/Serum: prealbumin, albumin, Ca, Fe, carotenes, Vit A, Ⓟ.
Additional tests for malabsorption include:

Schilling Test for Vit B$_{12}$ absorption
D-Xylose absorption

24-hour fecal fat
Tryptophan load test for Vit B$_6$

TESTS RELATED TO ETOH ABUSE

The following blood levels may be increased above the usual norm:
Blood/Serum: GGT, MCV, SGOT, Alk Phos, Uric Acid, HDL Cholesterol.
Reference: The Psychiatric Times, Vol. 5, #6, June, 1988.

COMPARISON OF HEIGHT-WEIGHT TABLES

Height	Metropolitan 1983 Weights for Ages 25–59		Gerontology Research Center Weight Range for Men and Women by Age (Years)				
	Men	Women	20–29	30–39	40–49	50–59	60–69
ft-in			lb				
4-10	. . .	100-131	84-111	92-119	99-127	107-135	115-142
4-11	. . .	101-134	87-115	95-123	103-131	111-139	119-147
5-0	. . .	103-137	90-119	98-127	106-135	114-143	123-152
5-1	123-145	105-145	93-123	101-131	110-140	118-148	127-157
5-2	125-148	108-144	96-127	105-136	113-144	122-153	131-163
5-3	127-151	111-148	99-131	108-140	117-149	126-158	135-168
5-4	129-155	114-152	102-135	112-145	121-154	130-163	140-173
5-5	131-159	117-156	106-140	115-149	125-159	134-168	144-179
5-6	133-163	120-160	109-144	119-154	129-164	138-174	148-184
5-7	135-167	123-164	112-148	122-159	133-169	143-179	153-190
5-8	137-171	126-167	116-153	126-163	137-174	147-184	158-196
5-9	139-175	129-170	119-157	130-168	141-179	151-190	162-201
5-10	141-179	132-173	122-162	134-173	145-184	156-195	167-207
5-11	144-183	135-176	126-167	137-178	149-190	160-201	172-213
6-0	147-187	. . .	129-171	141-183	153-195	165-207	177-219
6-1	150-192	. . .	133-176	145-188	157-200	169-213	182-225
6-2	153-197	. . .	137-181	149-194	162-206	174-219	187-232
6-3	157-202	. . .	141-186	153-199	166-212	179-225	192-238
6-4	. . .	. . .	144-191	157-205	171-218	184-231	197-244

From: *Environmental Nutrition*, Vol. II, #3, March 1988.

Values in this table are for height without shoes and weight without clothes.

The weight range is the weight for small frame at the lower limit and large frame at the upper limit.

Segmental Weights for Limbs

This information may be used to estimate body weight for patients with amputations.

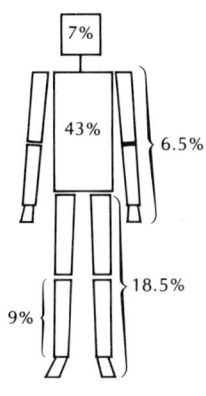

- Head: 7%
- Trunk: 43%
- Upper arm: 6.5%
- Thigh: 18.5%
- Lower leg: 9%

Reference
Reproduced with permission from Braune and Fischer in Brunnstrom, S.: Clinical Kinesiology. Philadelphia: F.A. Davis Co., 1972.

CALCULATION of DESIRABLE BODY WEIGHT

Build	Height	Calculation
Women:		
Medium Frame	1st 5 ft	Allow 100 lbs. & Add 5 lbs/inch
Large Frame		Add 10%
Small Frame		Subtract 10%
Men:		
Medium Frame	1st 5 ft	Allow 106 lbs & Add 6 lbs/inch
Large Frame		Add 10%
Small Frame		Subtract 10%

Handbook of Clinical Dietetics, Amer. Dietetic Assoc. p. 127, Yale University Press, 1981.
Davidson, J.K., Postgrad. Med. 59:114, 1976.

ADULT HEIGHT-WEIGHT RANGES 51 + YEARS

Females Height	Weight Range	Mean Weight	Males Height	Weight Range	Mean Weight
4'8"	81 - 99	90	5'0"	95-117	106
4'9"	83.5-102	92.5	5'1"	100-123	112
4'10"	85 -105	95	5'2"	106-130	118
4'11"	87.5-107	97.5	5'3"	111-136	124
5'0"	90 -110	100	5'4"	117-143	130
5'1"	94 -116	105	5'5"	122-150	136
5'2"	99 -121	110	5'6"	127-156	142
5'3"	104 -127	115	5'7"	133-163	148
5'4"	108 -132	120	5'8"	139-169	154
5'5"	112 -138	125	5'9"	144-176	160
5'6"	117 -143	130	5'10"	149-183	166
5'7"	121 -149	135	5'11"	154-189	172
5'8"	126 -154	140	6'0"	160-196	178
5'9"	130 -160	145	6'1"	166-202	184
5'10"	135 -165	150	6'2"	171-209	190

Reference: Healthcare Management Composite, Inc. 1987

CAFFEINE CONTENT OF SELECTED FOODS & BEVERAGES

Product	Caffeine Content (mg)
Beverages — mg/fl oz	Range
Roasted & ground	
percolated coffee	8 -34
drip coffee	11 -35
decaffeinated coffee	0.2- 0.4
Instant coffee	
decaffeinated	0.4- 1.6
instant, percolated & drip coffee	6 -35
Bagged tea	6 - 9
Leaf tea	6 -10
Instant tea	5 - 6
Cocoa	2 - 7

Soft Drinks — mg/fl oz	Range
Regular	
Cola or Pepper	2.5 -3.8
Decaffeinated Cola	trace -0.015
Lemon-Lime (clear)	0
Orange	0
Other Citrus	0 -4.5
Root Beer	0
Ginger Ale	0
Tonic Water	0
Other Regular	0 -3.6

Product	Caffeine Content (mg)
Food Products	Range
Chocolate Bar 30 g	4
Milk Chocolate 1 oz	1- 15
Sweet Chocolate	5- 35
Chocolate Milk 8 oz	2- 5
Baking Chocolate 1 oz	18-118

Soft Drinks — mg/fl oz	Range
Diet	
Diet Cola or Pepper	0.1 -4.9
Decaffeinated Diet Cola	trace -0.015
Diet Lemon-Lime	0
Diet Root Beer	0
Other Diets	0 -3.6
Club Soda, Seltzer, Sparkling Water	0

Caffeine, theophylline, and theobromine are xanthine derivatives.[4] Concurrent use may increase CNS stimulation and cause other additive toxic effects.[14]

Reference: 28

HERBAL TEAS: CAUTION

Potential Toxic Reactions from Certain Herbs.

Tonka beans, melilot, woodruff	Contains natural coumarins can cause coagulation defect
Foxglove, dogbane, lily-of-the-valley, oleander	Plants with digitalis-like activity can cause digitalis toxicity
Licorice tea in large quantities	Can cause sodium retention, potassium loss, diarrhea, elevated blood pressure
Chamomile	Allergies to marigold, yarrow, asters, ragweed, chrysanthemums can cause anaphylactic reactions
Senna, aloe, buckthorn, dock	Can cause severe diarrhea
Shave grass, horsetail	Can cause acute neurotoxicity
Comfrey	Contains hepatotoxic pyrrolizidine alkaloids
Sassafras	Contains a potent carcinogen: safrole
Burdock, catnip, juniper, hydrangea, jimson weed	Can induce bizarre anticholinergic effects

Most herb tea is rich in tannins which can complex with, inactivate, or prolong the absorption of certain drugs.

Some Herbs That Should Not Be Used in Foods, Beverages, or Drugs

Buckeyes, aesculus, horse chestnut	Contains a toxic coumarin glycoside

Mistletoe, viscum, American mistletoe	Contains the toxic pressor amines B-phenylethylamine and tyramine
Lily-of-the-valley, convallaria, May lily	Contains the toxic cardiac glycosides convallatoxin, convallarin, convallamarin
Periwinkle, vinca, greater periwinkle, lesser periwinkle	Contains toxic alkaloids vinblastine & vincristine: cytotoxic and neurological actions. Hepatotoxicity
Ginseng	Decreases serum glucose Increases cortisol

FOOD SOURCES OF OXALATES

Fruits	Vegetables	Nuts	Beverages
Blackberries	Asparagus	* Almonds	* Chocolate
Cranberries	Beans, green & wax	* Cashew nuts	* Cocoa
Currants	* Beets	* Pepper	Colas
Figs	* Beet greens	* Poppy seeds	
Gooseberries	* Chard		
Grapes, Concord	Endive		
Lemon Peel	* Lambsquarter		
Oranges	Okra		
Plums	* Parsley		
Raspberries, black	* Purslane		
Rhubarb	* Spinach		
* Strawberries	Sweet potato		
	Tomato		

* over 0.1% oxalic acid

PRESSOR AGENTS: TYRAMINE, DOPAMINE, PHENYLETHYLAMINE IN FOODS AND BEVERAGES

FOODS WHICH MUST BE AVOIDED: All cheeses including "imitation" (except fresh cottage, ricotta, cream). Chianti, vermouth wines, beer and ale: tyramine content variable. Smoked or pickled fish (herring), caviar, chopped liver, pate, other prepared non-fresh meats, dry or semi-dry sausages (pepperoni), beef tenderized or marinated over 24 hr, Fava or broad bean pods (Italian green beans contain dopamine), sauerkraut, Meat extracts, yeast extracts/brewer's yeast.

FOODS TO BE CONSUMED WITH CAUTION: Means small servings (½ cup/4oz or less).
Soups made with instant soup powders, or with meat bases of yeast extracts or miso. Kim chee. Soy sauce. Ripe avocado, banana. Yogurt, sour cream, acidophilus milk, buttermilk. Fresh raspberries. Peanuts. Chocolate. Red and white wines, distilled spirits.

FOODS WITH INSUFFICIENT EVIDENCE TO SUPPORT EXCLUSION: Yeast breads, coffee, tea and caffeine containing beverages, fresh pineapple, salad dressing, raisins, tomato juice, canned figs, anchovies, Worcestershire sauce.

1. The tyramine content varies from product to product and even between samples of the same product. The portion of cheese closer to the rind has a much higher tyramine content than the portion farthest away. Consumption of 6mg of tyramine may produce some degree of hypertension while 10–25mg can lead to a more severe crisis. The amount a person eats will determine the total dose of tyramine consumed, e.g., as little as 1oz of cheddar cheese yielding 15–45mg could cause a moderate to severe hypertensive action.
2. Use care when eating out: Choose plainer dishes rather than casseroles or dishes with sauces.
3. Caffeine, a weak pressor agent, in excessive amounts could possibly produce symptoms unrelated to tyramine content.

4. The tyramine content generally increases with the aging process; any protein rich food may undergo protein degradation given contamination and sufficient storage time. Cooking of degraded protein does not destroy the tyramine content. Recommend: perishable refrigerated items be consumed within 48 hr of purchase.
5. Patients have been known to eat tyramine containing foods on occasion without adverse effect, but there is no guarantee that the same foods will not produce a severe reaction in the future.

Reference: 36, 21

HISTAMINE: Foods highest are fish (such as tuna, sardines, skipjack) that have started to spoil, even before any change in taste is perceptible.

PATIENT COUNSELING*

- Obtain a good dietary history, questioning use of specific foods, amounts, and frequency.
- Evaluate probability of patient adherence to the diet on the basis of the degree of change necessary in his food habits and *not* on his intelligence, educational level, etc.
- Be very specific about the foods to be avoided and the consequences of nonadherence.
- Have all health professionals involved in the patient's care knowledgeable *and* in consensus about the dietary restrictions.
- Review diet and evaluate dietary adherence on a regular basis by asking specific dietary questions.

* From: Tsuang & McCabe reference.

GOITROGENIC FOODS

May cause hypothyroidism or goiter unless dietary iodine is sufficient

Asparagus	Cabbage	Soy Beans	Spinach
Broccoli	Kale	Lettuce	Turnip Greens
Brussels Sprouts	Other leafy, green vegetables	Peas	Watercress

References: VanDerlinde, L.: Drug, food, drink interactions. Amer. J. Hosp. Pharm. 26:107,1969
Pierpaoli, P.: Drug Therapy and diet. Drug Intell. and Clinical Pharm 6:6:89, 1972
Lambert, M.: Drug and diet interactions. Am. J. Nursing 75:403, 1975

VITAMIN K (mcg) IN SELECTED FOODS AND BEVERAGES

Item	Mean	Range	Item	Mean	Range
BEVERAGES			**VEGETABLES**		
coffee — 6 fl oz (180g)	68		asparagus, raw — 5–6 spears (100g)	57	
tea, green — 8 fl oz (240g)	1709		broccoli, raw — 1 cup (126g)	252	
FATS			brussels sprouts, raw — 3½oz (100g)		800–3000
oil, corn — 3½oz (100g)	50		cabbage, raw — 1 cup (124g)	155	
oil, soybean — 3½oz (100g)	500		cauliflower, raw — 3½oz (100g)	3600	
MEAT			green beans, raw — 3½oz (100g)	290	
beef, ground, ckd — 3½oz (100g)	7		lettuce, raw — 1 cup (74g)	95	
beef, ground, ckd, gamma-irradiated			peas, green, unripe — 3½oz (100g)	300	
— 3½oz (100g)	0		peas, green, boiled — ½cup (85g)	221	
beef, liver, raw — 3½oz (100g)	92		potato, raw — 3½oz (100g)	80	
liverwurst — 1oz (28g)	34		spinach, raw — 3½oz (100g)	89	40–3000
MILK			tomato, raw — 1 med (148g)	7	
cow milk, whole — 1 liter	60		turnip greens, raw — 1 cup (54g)	351	
human milk — 1 liter	15		watercress, raw — 25 sprigs (25g)	14	

From: Pennington & Church, *Bowes & Church's Food Values of Portions Commonly Used*, 1985.

TABULATION OF pH AND ACID CONTENT OF VARIOUS BEVERAGES
(In order of decreasing acid content)

	pH	mEq acid/cc		pH	mEq acid/cc
Vinegar (cider)	3.1-3.2	0.60-.64	Ginger ale (can)	2.7-2.9	0.041-.054
Grapefruit juice	3.5	0.15-.17	Club soda	3.7	0.046
Pineapple juice	3.4-3.5	0.13-.14	Peach nectar	3.6	0.038-.039
Orange juice	3.4-3.8	0.12-.13	Prune juice	4.1-4.2	0.031-.036
Grape juice	3.3-3.4	0.056-.096	Pear nectar	3.7	0.021-.022
Cranberry juice	2.6-2.8	0.080-.081	Skim milk	6.5-6.7	0.007-.009
Diet cola (can) (Tab)	2.9	0.042	Half & Half cream	6.6-6.7	0.005-.007
(Open 1 Hr.)	2.9-3.1	0.057-.082	Whole milk	6.6-6.7	0.005-.006
Apricot nectar	3.8	0.055-.062	Coffee (whole)	4.9-5.1	0.004-.006
Orange soda	2.8	0.056-.058	Sanka (instant)	5.1-5.4	0.004-.005
Orange drink	2.6	0.055	Cocoa (instant)	6.7-6.9	0.001-.002
Apple juice	3.5-3.6	0.053-.056	Tea (instant)	6.8-6.9	0.001
Tomato juice	4.3	0.049-.059	Tap water	7.6-8.2	—
7-Up	3.0-3.1	0.048-.055			

From: Flick, A. L., University Hospital, San Diego, CA, "Digestive Diseases" 15:317-320, 1970. Article entitled — Acid Content of Common Beverages.

	pH of Coke		pH of Coke
Old ("Classic") Coke	2.38	New Coke — caffeine-free	2.25
New Coke	2.37	Diet Coke	2.89

From: New Eng. Jr. Med. 11/21/85 pg. 1351

FOODS POTENTIALLY CAUSING CHANGES IN URINARY pH

Potentially Acid or Acid-Ash Foods

Meat	Meat; fish; fowl; shellfish; eggs; all types of cheese; peanut butter; peanuts
Fat	Bacon; nuts (Brazil nuts, filberts, walnuts)
Starch	All types of bread (especially whole wheat), cereals, and crackers; macaroni; spaghetti; noodles; rice
Vegetable	Corn; lentils
Fruit	Cranberries; plums; prunes
Dessert	Plain cakes; cookies

Potentially Basic or Alkaline-Ash Foods

Milk	Milk and milk products; cream; buttermilk
Fat	Nuts (almonds, chestnuts, coconut)
Vegetable	All types (except corn, lentils), especially beets, beet greens, Swiss chard, dandelion greens, kale, mustard greens, spinach, turnip greens
Fruit	All types (except cranberries, prunes, plums)
Sweets	Molasses

Neutral Foods

Fats	Butter; margarine; cooking fats; oils
Sweets	Plain candies; sugar; syrup; honey
Starch	Arrowroot; corn; tapioca
Beverages	Coffee; tea

INDICATIONS AND RATIONALE

Description of foods as either "acid-ash" or "alkaline-ash" is based on the reaction of the ash remaining after combustion of foods under laboratory conditions. Acid-ash foods tend to promote a more acidic urine. Conversely, alkaline-ash foods tend to promote a more alkaline urine.

A strict dietary regimen is rarely necessary. Since diet is generally considered an auxiliary measure to acidifying or alkalinizing medications, simply avoiding excessive use of particular foods may be sufficient. For example, if medical treatment is directed at acidifying the urine, the diet should not contain large amounts of alkaline-ash foods; complete avoidance of all alkaline-ash foods, however, would probably not yield any further benefit and is unwarranted.

From: *Mayo Clinic Diet Manual*, 1981

SALT SUBSTITUTES

Brand	Potassium Content
Adolph's	2340mg/ 5gm
Adolph's Seasoned	1328mg/ 5gm
Morton	2736mg/ 5gm
Morton Seasoned	2100mg/ 5gm
Nosalt	1368mg/2.5gm
Neocurtasal	2340mg/ 5gm
Nu-salt	2640mg/ 5gm
Morton Lite Salt	1466mg/ 5gm
Lawry's Seasoned Salt Free	1160mg/ 5gm

Reference: Russell, "Potassium supplementation, K-retaining diuretics, and hyperkalemia," Journal of Clinical Nutrition, Vol. 6 #2, March/April 1987.

PHYSICAL SIGNS OF MALNUTRITION

Body Area	Signs	Possible Causes
Hair	Dull, dry: lack of natural shine;	Protein-Calorie deficiency
	Thin, sparse; loss of curl;	Zinc deficiency
	Color changes; easily plucked	Other nutrient deficiencies: Mn,
	Depigmentation	Cu
Eyes	Small, yellowish lumps around eyes; White rings around both eyes	Hyperlipidemia
	Pale eye membranes	Vit B_{12}, Folacin and/or Fe deficiency
	Night blindness, dry membranes, dull or soft cornea	Vit A, Zn deficiency
	Redness & fissures of eyelid corners	Niacin deficiency
	Angular inflammation of eyelids	Riboflavin deficiency
	Ring of fine blood vessels around cornea	General poor nutrition
Lips	Redness & swelling of mouth	Niacin, Riboflavin, Fe and/or B_6 deficiency
	Angular fissures, scars at corner of mouth	
Gums	Spongy, swelling, bleed easily, redness	Vit C deficiency
	Gingivitis	Vit A, Niacin, Riboflavin deficiency
Mouth	Cheilosis, angular scars	Riboflavin, Folic acid deficiency
Tongue	Sores, swollen, scarlet & raw	Folacin, Niacin, deficiency
	Smooth with Papillae (small projections)	Riboflavin, Vit B_{12}, Pyridoxine, Fe, or Zn deficiency
	Glossitis	
	Purplish color	Riboflavin deficiency

Taste	Sense of taste diminished	Zinc deficiency
Teeth	Gray-brown spots	Increased fluoride intake
	Missing or erupting abnormally	General poor nutrition
Face	Skin color loss; dark cheeks & eyes; enlarged parotid glands, scaling of skin around nostrils	Protein-Calorie deficiency. Niacin, Riboflavin, & Pyridoxine deficiencies specifically.
	Pallor	Fe, Folacin, Vit B_{12}, & Vit C deficiencies
	Hyperpigmentation	Niacin deficiency
Neck	Thyroid enlargement	Iodine deficiency
	Symptoms of hypothyroidism	
Nails	Fragility, banding	Protein deficiency
	Spoon-shaped	Fe deficiency
Skin	Slow wound healing	Zinc deficiency
	Psoriasis	Biotin deficiencies
	Scaliness	Biotin deficiency
	Black & blue marks due to skin bleeding	Vit C and/or Vit K deficiency
	Dryness, mosaic, sandpaper feel, flakiness of skin	Vit A increased or decreased
	Swollen & dark	Niacin deficiency
	Lack of fat under skin, bilateral edema	Protein-Calorie deficiency
	Yellow-colored	Carotene deficiency/excess
	Cutaneous flushing	Niacin
	Pallor	Fe, Folic acid deficiency

PHYSICAL SIGNS OF MALNUTRITION

Body Area	Signs	Possible Causes
Gastro-Intestinal	Anorexia, flatulence, diarrhea	B_{12} deficiency
Muscular System	Weakness	Phosphorus or Potassium deficiency
	Wasted appearance	Protein-Calorie deficiency
	Calf tenderness; absent knee-jerks	Thiamin deficiency
	Peripheral neuropathy	Folacin, Pyridoxine, Pantothenic acid, Phosphate, Thiamin deficiencies
	Muscle twitching	Magnesium or Pyridoxine excesses/deficiency
	Muscle cramps	Chloride decreased, Sodium deficiency
	Muscle pain	Biotin deficiency
Skeletal System	Demineralization of bone	Ca, P deficiencies; Vit D deficiency
	Epiphyseal enlargement of leg & knee	Vit D deficiency
	Bowed legs	Vit D deficiency
	Growth failure in children	Protein, Vit D deficiency
Nervous System	Listlessness	Protein-Calorie deficiency
	Loss of position & vibratory sense; decrease & loss of ankle & knee reflexes	Thiamin & Vit B_{12} deficiency
	Seizures, memory impairment & behavioral disturbances	Magnesium deficiency; Zinc deficiency
	Peripheral neuropathy, dementia	Pyr deficiency

References: Barness, Coble, Macdonald, Christakis. *Nutrition in Medical Practice*. Westport: AVI Publishing, 1981.

Christakis, G. ed. "Nutritional Assessment in Health Programs." *American Journal of Public Health*. 63: Supplement No. 1 (Nov) 1973.

Paige. *Manual of Clinical Nutrition*. New Jersey: NPI, 1983.

REFERENCES

1. AMA Drug Evaluations, 6th Edition, American Medical Assoc. (Chicago, IL, American Medical Assoc., 1988).
2. Handbook of Nonprescription Drugs, 7th Edition, American Pharmaceutical Assoc. (Washington, D.C., Amer. Pharmaceutical Assoc., 1982).
3. Compendium of Drug Therapy, Biomedical Information Corp. (New York City, NY, Biomedical Information Corp., 1987-1988).
4. Gilman, A.G., Goodman, L.S., Rall, T.W., & Murad, F., The Pharmacological Basis of Therapeutics, 7th Edition (New York City, NY, Macmillan, 1985).
5. Hansten, P.D., PharmD, Drug Interactions, 5th Edition (Philadelphia, PA, Lea & Febiger, 1985).
6. Hathcock, J.N. & Coon, J., Nutrition and Drug Interrelations (New York City, NY, Academic Press, 1978).
7. Facts and Comparisons, Kastrup, E.K., BS Pharm.: Editor (St. Louis, MO, J.B. Lippincott Co., 1988).
8. Martin, E.W., Hazards of Medications (Philadelphia, PA, J.B. Lippincott Co., 1971).
9. "The Medical Letter on Drugs and Therapeutics," (New Rochelle, NY, Vol. 22-30, Issue 766, 1988).
10. Physicians Desk Reference, 42nd Edition (Oradell, NJ, Medical Economics Co., 1988).
11. Roe, D.A., MD
    Drug-Induced Nutritional Deficiencies (Westport, CT, The Avi Publishing Co., 1976).
    Geriatric Nutrition (Englewood Cliffs, NJ, Prentice-Hall, Inc., 1983)
    Handbook: Interactions of Selected Drugs and Nutrients in the Patient, Third Edition (Chicago, IL, American Dietetic Assoc., 1982).
    "Therapeutic Effects of Drug-Nutrient Interactions in the Elderly," JADA, Vol. 85, #2, p. 174, 1985.
    Drugs & Nutrition in the Geriatric Patient, Editor (New York City, Churchill-Livingston, 1985).
    et al, "Effects of Fiber Supplements on Apparent Absorption of Pharmacological Doses of Riboflavin," JADA, Vol. 88, #2, p. 211, 1988.
12. Schneider, H.A., PhD, Anderson, C.E., PhD, Coursin, D.B., Nutritional Support of Medical Practice (Hagerstown, MD, Medical Dept., Harper & Row, 1977).
13. United States Pharmacopeia Dispensing Information, 8th Edition
    Vol. I Drug Information for the Health Provider
    Vol. II Advice for the Patient
    (Rockville, MD, USP Convention, 1988)

14. Smith, C.H., RD, PhD: Editor, "Dietary Concerns Associated with the Use of Medications," *JADA*, Vol. 84, #8, p. 901, 1984.

15. Morgan, B.L.G., PhD, <u>The Food and Drug Interaction Guide</u> (New York City, NY, Simon and Schuster, Inc., 1986).

16. *Handbook of Clinical Dietetics*, American Dietetic Assoc. (New Haven/London, Yale University Press, 1981).

17. *American Journal of Nursing* (New York City, 1981–1987).

18. "Effect of Food on Drug Bio-Availability," *Annual Review of Pharmacological Toxicology*, Vol. 20:173, 1980.

19. Bezchlibnyk, K.Z., Director of Pharmacy, Clarke Institute of Psychiatry, Toronto, Ontario, Canada, "Should Psychiatric Patients Drink Coffee?", *Canadian Medical Assoc. Journal*, Vol. 124: 4, Feb. 15, 1981.

20. Smith, C.H., RD, PhD & Bidlack, W.R., PhD
    "Food and Drug Interactions," *Food Technology*, October, 1982, p. 99–103.
    "Effect of Nutritional Factors on Hepatic Drug & Toxicant Metabolism," *JADA*, Vol. 84, #8, p. 892, 1984.

21. *Biological Therapies in Psychiatry*, Massachusetts General Hospital Newsletter, PSG-Wright, Inc., Littleton, MA, March, 1981–June, 1988.

22. Carr, C.J., "Food and Drug Interactions," *Annual Review of Pharmacology Toxicology*, Vol. 22:19–29, 1982.

23. Chaplin, S., Sanders, G.L., Smith, J.M., "Drugs Excretion in Human Breast Milk," *Adv. Drug React. AC Poison Review*, Vol. 1:4, p. 255–287, October, 1982.

24. Christakis, G.: Editor, "Nutritional Assessment in Health Programs," *American Journal of Public Health* — 63:Supplement No. 1, Nov., 1973.

25. *Dairy Council Digest*, Rosemont, IL, National Dairy Council, March–April, 1980 thru March–April, 1988 (Vol. 59, #2).

26. "FDA's Drug Review Process is Focus of Attention in 1987," *American Journal of Hospital Pharmacy*, Vol. 45, p. 446, March, 1988.

27. *Drug Therapy*, Biomedical Information Corp., New York City, NY, 1981–1985.

28. *FDA Consumer*, US Dept of Health Services, Rockville, MD, 1983–1988.

29. Norwich-Eaton Pharmaceuticals, Inc., *RD — Essential News for Dietitians*, Vol. 4–8.

30. Lamy, P.P., PhD
    "How Your Patients' Diet Can Affect Drug Response," *Drug Therapy*, Vol. 10:8:82–90, August, 1980.
    "Effects of Diet and Nutrition on Drug Therapy," *Journal of the American Geriatric Society*, supplement to Vol. 30:11, p. 99, 1982.
    "A Consideration of NSAID Use in the Elderly," *Geriatric Medicine Today*, Vol. 7, #4, April, 1988.

31. Dalton-Bunnow, M.F., "Sulfite Content of Drug Products," *American Journal of Hospital Pharmacy*, Vol. 42, p. 2195-2201, October, 1985.
32. University of Alabama Hospitals, *Practical Guide to Nutritional Care*, Birmingham, AL, 1984.
33. Fish, K.H., Jr, PharmD, & Pearson, R.E., MS, *Sodium Content of Selected Medicinals*, Michigan Regional Drug Information Network & Michigan Heart Assoc., a pamphlet, 1968.
34. *Nutrition & the MD*, Van Nuys, CA, PM, Inc., Vol. V-XIV, 1988.
35. *Nutrition Research Newsletter*, LYDA Associates, Palisades, NY, thru 1988.
36. *Currents in Affective Illness*, Editor: Rosenblatt, J.E. MD & Rosenblatt, N., MD, Vol. V, #2, Feb. 1986 thru Vol. VII, #5, May, 1988.
37. Haas, E., PharmD, & Lemmons, A., "Drug-Induced Taste Disorders," *Current Concepts in Hospital Pharmacy Management*, p. 16, Summer, 1988.
38. Grant, A., MS, RD & DeHoog, S., RD, *Nutritional Assessment and Support*, 3rd Edition, p. 23-124 (Seattle, WA, Grant & DeHoog, 1985).
39. Menon, I.S., Kendal, R.Y., Dewar, H.A., & Newell, D.J., "Effect of Onions on Blood Fibrinolytic Activity," *British Medical Journal*, 3:351, 1968.
40. *JCAH Accreditation Manual for Hospitals, Standard IV*, Chicago, IL, American Hospital Assoc., 1984.
41. *Archives of Internal Medicine*
    Vol. 144, p. 710, April, 1984.
    Vol. 147, Sept./Oct., 1987.
    Vol. 148, Jan., 1988, Cholesterol Adult Treatment Panel.
42. *The Psychiatric Times*, Vol. V, #6, June, 1988.
43. Emerson, A.P., MS, RD, "Foods High in Fiber and Phytobezoar Formation," *JADA*, Vol. 87, #12, p. 1675, Dec, 1987.
44. Wallach, J., MD, *Interpretation of Diagnostic Tests*, 4th Edition (Boston/Toronto, Little, Brown and Company, 1986), Chapter 13.
45. *Harrison's Principles of Internal Medicine*, 10th Edition, Editors: Petersdorf, R.G., MD, et al (New York, NY, McGraw-Hill Book Company, 1983).

ADDITIONAL REFERENCES

American Druggist, "Top 200 Prescription Drugs of 1987," Feb., 1988.

Aspects of Aging, Unit I — Psychological Issues #1–6; Unit II — Physiologic Issues #1–3, Continuing Education Service, Smith, Kline & French Laboratories, Philadelphia, PA, 1985.

Betterley, C., Schafer, E., & Nelson, D., "Food-Drug Interactions," A Slide & VCR Tape Set with Teaching Kit. Iowa State Univ. — Coop Extension Service, Ames, IA, 1986.

Bosso, J.A., Pharm.D. & Pearson, R.E., MS, "Sugar Content of Selected Liquid Medicinals," *Diabetes*, Vol. 22, #10, p. 776.

Clinical Report on Aging, American Geriatric Society, Vol. 2, #2, p. 18, 1988.

Current Concepts in Hospital Pharmacy Management, Summer, 1988, p. 16.

Dietetic Currents, Editor: Gussler, J.D., PhD, Ross Laboratories, Columbus, OH, thru Vol. 15 #3, 1988.

<u>Dorland's Illustrated Medical Dictionary</u>, 25th Edition (Philadelphia, PA, W.B. Saunders, 1974).

Drug Abuse & Alcoholism Newsletter, Editor: Cohen, S., MD, Vista Hill Foundation, San Diego, CA, thru Vol. XVII, #5, June, 1988. Schuckit, M., MD (new Editor), "A Prediction of Outcome Among Alcoholics," Vol. XVII, #4, May 1988.

"Drug and Nutrient Interaction Slide Program & Reference Chart," Mead-Johnson Nutritional Division, Evansville, IN, 1986.

Dwyer, J., DSc, RD, Foulkes, E., MS, RD, Evans, M., MS, RD & Ausman, L., DSc, RD, "Acid/alkaline ash diets: Time for assessment and change," *JADA*, Vol. 85, #7, July, 1985.

Environmental Nutrition, New York City, NY, thru Vol. 11, #5, 1988.

Flick, A.L., "Acid Content of Common Beverages," *Digestive Diseases*, 15:317–320, 1970. University Hospital, San Diego, CA.

Frisancho, A.R., PhD
  "New Standards of Weight and Body Composition by Frame Size and Height for Assessment of Nutritional Status of Adults and the Elderly," *American Journal of Clinical Nutrition*, Vol. 40, p. 808, October, 1984.
  "Nutritional Anthropometry," *JADA*, Vol. 88, #5, May, 1988.

Geriatric Medicine Today, Plainsboro, NJ, Med Publishing Inc. thru Vol. 7, #6, June, 1988.

Hamilton, E.M.N., & Gropper, S.A.S., The Biochemistry of Human Nutrition (St. Paul, MN, West Publishing Company, 1987).

Hamilton, E.N., & Whitney, E.M.N., Understanding Nutrition, 3rd Edition (St. Paul, MN, West Publishing Company, 1984).

Harper, S., MS, RD & Higgins, W., PhD, "Oral Antibiotics and Meal Interference in Kentucky Hospitals," Dept. of Health and Safety, Western Kentucky University, Bowling Green, KY, 1984.

Harshorn, E.A., "Food and Drug Interactions," JADA, Vol. 70, p. 15, 1977.

Harvard Medical School Health Letter, Cambridge, MA, thru May 1988.

Hospital Pharmacy, New York City, NY, Biomedical Information Corp, 1984-1988.

Journal of the American Dietetic Association (JADA), Chicago, IL, American Dietetic Assoc., 1976-1988.

Journal of Clinical Psychiatry, Memphis, TN, Physicians Post-graduate Press, Inc., thru Vol. 49, #5, May, 1988.

Journal of Nutrition Education, Oakland, CA, Society for Nutrition Education, thru Vol. 20, #3, June, 1988.

Journal of Nutrition for the Elderly, Editor: Natow, A.B., PhD, Binghamton, NY, The Haworth Press, Inc.

Krupp, M.A., MD & Chatton, M.J., MD, Current Medical Diagnosis & Treatment (Los Altos, CA, Lange Medical Publications, 1975).

McCabe, B.J., PhD, RD & Tsuang, M., "Dietary Considerations in MAOI Regimens," J. of Clinical Psychiatry, 43:5:177, 1982.

"Dietary Tyramine and Other Pressor Amines in MAOI Regimens: a Review," JADA, Vol. 86, #8, August, 1986.

& Blackwell, B., MD, "MAOI — Food Interactions," Currents in Affective Illness, Vol. 7, #4, April, 1988.

Manual of Clinical Nutrition, Editor: Paige, D.M., MD, MPH (Pleasantville, NY, Nutrition Publications, Inc., 1983) & Updates.

Mayo Clinic Diet Manual, Philadelphia, PA, W.B. Saunders, 1981.

Miller, S.A., Nutrition and Behavior (Philadelphia, PA, Franklin Institute Press, 1981).

Modern Medicine, "Herbal Teas Linked with Digitalis Toxicity," Nov-Dec, 1980.

National Academy of Sciences (NRC), 1980 Recommended Dietary Allowances, 9th Edition, Washington, DC.

National Soft Drink Assoc., "What's in Soft Drinks?", Washington, DC, Sept. 1982.

New England Journal of Medicine, Boston, MA, Massachusetts Medical Society, Vol. 308-318.

Nutrition and Health, Institute of Human Nutrition, Columbia University, New York City, Vol. 3, #6 thru Vol. 10, #1.

Nutrition, Food & Aging, California Dept of Aging, Sacramento, CA, thru Vol. 8 #III, 1988.

<u>Nutrition and Medical Practice</u>, Editors: Barness, L.A., MD, Coble, Y.D., Jr., MD, Macdonald, D.I., MD, & Christakis, G., PhD (Westport, CT, AVI Publishing Company, Inc., 1981).

<u>PDR for Non-Prescription Drugs</u>, 8th Edition (Oradell, NJ, Medical Economics Co., Inc., 1987).

Pennington, J.A.T., PhD & Church, H.N., BS, <u>Bowes & Church's Food Values of Portions Commonly Used</u>, 14th Edition (Philadelphia, PA, J.B. Lippincott Company, 1985).

Psychosomatics, Academy of Psychosomatic Medicine, Greenwich, CT, Cliggott Publishing Co., Vol. 28, #2, thru May, 1988.

Psychiatric Annals, Journal of Continuing Psychiatric Education, Thorofare, NJ, SLACK, Inc., thru Vol. 18, #6, June, 1988.

Randle, N.W., BS, RPh, "Food or Nutrient Effects on Drug Absorption — A Review," *Hospital Pharmacy*, Vol. 22, July, 1987.

Raymond, G., RPh, MS, Day, P., RPh & Rabb, M., RPh, MS, "Sodium Content of Commonly Administered Intravenous Drugs," *Hospital Pharmacy*, Vol. 17, #10, p. 560, October, 1982.

Resident & Staff Physician, Port Washington, NY, The Resident, Inc., 1983–1988.

Ross Laboratories, *Nutritional Screening and Assessment as Components of Hospital Admission*, Report of the 8th Ross Round Table on Medical Issues, held June, 1987, Dallas, Texas.

Russell, R., MD, "Potassium supplementation, K-retaining diuretics and hyperkalemia," *Clinical Nutrition*, Vol. 6, #2, March/April 1987.

Sauberlich, H.E., Dowdy, R.P. & Skala, J.H., <u>Laboratory Test for the Assessment of Nutritional Status</u> (Boca Raton, FL, CRC Press, Inc., 1981).

Shils, M.E., MD, ScD & Young, V.R., PhD, <u>Modern Nutrition in Health and Disease</u>, 7th Edition (Philadelphia, PA, Lea & Febiger, 1988).

Souney, P.F., Cyr, D.A., Chang, J.T. & Kaul, A.E., "Sugar Content of Selected Pharmaceuticals," *Diabetes Care*, Vol. 6, #3, p. 231, May–June, 1983.

"Suggested Guidelines for Nutrition Management of the Critically Ill Patient," Quality Assurance Committee, Dietitians in Critical Care Dietetic Practice Group, American Dietetic Assoc., Chicago, IL, 1984.

Toothaker, R.D. & Welling, P.G., "The Effect of Food on Drug Bio-availability," *Annual Review of Pharmacology Toxicology*, Vol. 20:173–199, 1980.

Tufts University, *Diet and Nutrition Newsletter*, thru Vol. 6, #3, May, 1988.

Walczak, R., MPH, "Identifying Adverse Drug Reactions and Food-Drug Interactions," *QRC Advisor*, Vol. 2, #9, July, 1986.

Weibert, R.T., PharmD & Norcross, W.A., MD, *Drug Interactions Index*, 2nd Edition (Oradell, NJ, Medical Economics Books, 1988).

Weller, R.A., MD & Preskorn, S.H., MD, "Psychotropic Drugs and Alcohol: Pharmacokinetic and Pharmacodynamic Interactions," *Psychosomatics*, Vol. 25, #4, p. 301, April, 1984.

Yamanaka-Yuen, N.A., PharmD, "Ethanol & Drug Interactions," *Drug Interactions Newsletter*, Vol. 5, #11, Nov., 1985.

ORDER FORM

Send book(s) to:

Name _____

Address _____

City _____ State _____ Zip _____

PRICES:

    1 @ $ 9.95 each
    2 @ $19.90
  3–10 @ $ 8.95 each
11–20 @ $ 8.25 each
21–30 @ $ 7.55 each
31–50 @ $ 6.85 each
51–100 @ $ 6.50 each

Price includes postage & handling.

Quantity _____ @ $ _____

TOTAL ENCLOSED _____

PREPAYMENT REQUIRED.
PLEASE PAY IN U.S. FUNDS.
OUTSIDE U.S.A., SEND ADDITIONAL $1.00/BOOK.
ALLOW 4–6 WEEKS FOR DELIVERY.

FOOD MEDICATION INTERACTIONS

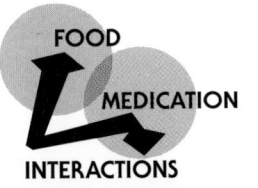

Enclose with your check or money order in an envelope.

MAIL TO:
FOOD-MEDICATION INTERACTIONS
P.O. Box 44033   or   P.O. Box 26464
Phoenix, Arizona 85064   Tempe, Arizona 85285